# A Colour Atlas of Oral Pathology

Copyright © K. W. Lee, 1985
Published by Wolfe Medical Publications Ltd, 1985
Printed by Royal Smeets Offset b.v., Weert, Netherlands
ISBN 0 7234 0807 6 Cased edition
ISBN 0 7234 1601 X Paperback edition
Paperback edition © 1989

For a full list of Wolfe Medical Atlases, plus
forthcoming titles and details of our surgical,
dental and veterinary Atlases, please write to
Wolfe Publishing Ltd, 2-16 Torrington Place,
London WC1E 7LT.

General Editor, Wolfe Medical Atlases:
G. Barry Carruthers, MD(Lond)

All rights reserved. No reproduction, copy or transmission
of this publication may be made without written permission.

No paragraph of this publication may be reproduced, copied
or transmitted save with written permission or in accordance
with the provisions of the Copyright Act 1956 (as amended),
or under the terms of any licence permitting limited copying
issued by the Copyright Licensing Agency,
33-34 Alfred Place, London WC1E 7DP.

Any person who does any unauthorised act in relation to
this publication may be liable to criminal prosecution and
civil claims for damages.

A CIP catalogue record for this book
is available from the British Library.

# A Colour Atlas of
# Oral Pathology

**K W Lee**     MDS, FDSRCS, FRC Path.

Reader in Oral Pathology, University of London,
Head of Department of Pathology,
Institute of Dental Surgery,
Eastman Dental Hospital, London,
Visiting Professor in Oral Pathology,
National University of Singapore

Wolfe Medical Publications Ltd

To Ivor R. H. Kramer OBE
who first unravelled for me
the mysteries of oral pathology

# Contents

# Acknowledgements

I am deeply grateful to my predecessor, Professor I. R. H. Kramer who founded the Department of Pathology, Eastman Dental Hospital in 1949, and built-up the collection of material from which most of the photomicrographs in this Atlas have been prepared. I must especially acknowledge the use of figures 152, 153, 154, 155, 156, 157, 158, 159, 160 and 256. Most of the sections were prepared by Mr A. Smith, Senior Chief Medical Laboratory Scientific Officer, and the technical staff of the department.

To Dr G.C. Blake, I am indebted for figures 133, 134, 135, 136, 426; to Professor G.B. Winter, for figure 194; Dr F.A.C. Oehlers of Singapore for figure 215; the late Mr L.W. Kay for figure 305; Mr A.E. Acosta for figures 65 and 69; Dr D.E.R. Cornick for figure 24; Mr V.J. Ward for figure 212; Professor D.H. Wright for providing the section for figure 376; Dr M. B. Edwards for figures 374, 464 and 465; Dr H. K. Thomsen, Copenhagen for figure 366; Dr L. Crome for figure 462; Dr W. K. Yip of Singapore for figure 339. The permission of the Editor, British Dental Journal, to use figure 285; the Editor, Cancer, to use figure 268; Pergamon Press Ltd to use figures 236 and 264 (from *The Periodontal Ligament in Health and Disease*, Berkowitz/Moxham/Newman) is gratefully acknowledged.

Miss Melanie Willingham and Miss Stephanie Lee deserve my especial thanks for typing and retyping numerous drafts of the manuscript.

# Introduction

It used to be said 'As is your pathology, so is your practice'. Yet with the advancement of knowledge on all fronts in dentistry, it becomes increasingly difficult for the dental student to acquire an insight of the cellular basis of disease with the limited time at his disposal. This Atlas has been planned, therefore, to aid the student to acquire an understanding of oral pathology, to see how histopathology can be related to a clinical problem that the budding dental surgeon has to handle. The inclusion of some clinical and radiographic material has been deliberate, to remind the student that histopathology is but one of the parts of the elephant, and that he or she must attempt at all times to see the elephant as a whole.

While the Atlas caters mainly for undergraduate students, I hope that postgraduates preparing for one of the fellowship diplomas of the Royal Colleges will find it of assistance to them in the oral pathological segments of the examinations; trainee oral pathologists also should derive some benefit from it. Many of the clinical conditions referred to can be found in the Atlases that form part of the series of books produced by the publisher, and the student is urged to correlate the information in these companion volumes with the information provided here, which is necessarily brief.

Magnifications have not been stated, as I believe that they are of little value, particularly when built-in landmarks such as blood cells are included. Unless otherwise stated, all sections are haematoxylin and eosin stained.

# 1 Lesions of the oral mucosa

## (i) Cells and normal structures

**1 Non-keratinized stratified squamous epithelium (cheek).** This type of epithelium covers a large part of the lining mucosa of the mouth, principally the cheeks, lips, floor of mouth and soft palate. It consists of a basal layer, a prickle-cell layer which forms the greater part of the thickness of the epithelium, and a few layers of flattened surface cells. Beneath the epithelium is the connective tissue of the lamina propria.

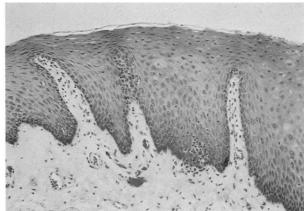

**2 Keratinized stratified squamous epithelium (hard palate).** This covers the hard palate, gingiva and the dorsal surface of the tongue. A thin layer of pink-stained keratin is seen on the surface.

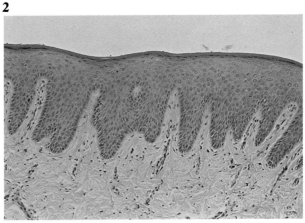

**3 Keratinized stratified squamous epithelium (tongue).** This covers the dorsal surface of the tongue but here the appearance is further modified by the presence of the lingual papillae.

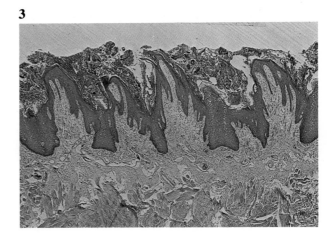

**4 Taste bud within the covering epithelium of the tongue.** The epithelium is parakeratinized, and a taste bud is present in the central area.

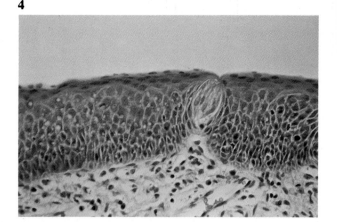

**5 Pseudostratified ciliated columnar epithelium.** This is the epithelium that lines the maxillary antrum and other parts of the respiratory tract. It is seen occasionally lining cysts of the oral tissues.

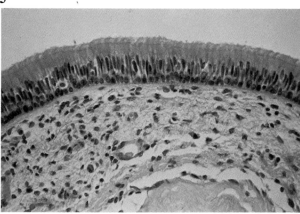

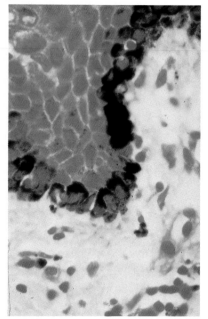

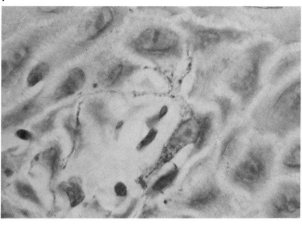

**6 Heavily pigmented gingival epithelium.** The basal cells of the epithelium are heavily pigmented with melanin. This patient is dark-skinned and the pigment is in both the melanocytes and the keratinocytes. *(Masson–Fontana)*

**7 Dendritic melanocyte.** It is not often that dendritic melanocytes can be made out in the basal cell region of the epithelium. They usually appear as clear cells. Here a dendritic melanocyte and its processes can be seen.

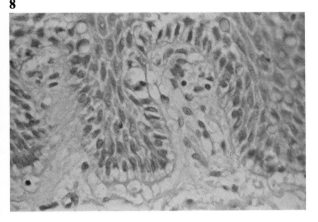

**8 Basement membrane.** The 'basement membrane' in light microscopy cannot be visualised in the vast majority of haematoxylin-eosin stained paraffin sections. Here a special stain, periodic acid Schiff method, has been used and the 'basement membrane' is seen as a magenta-coloured line.

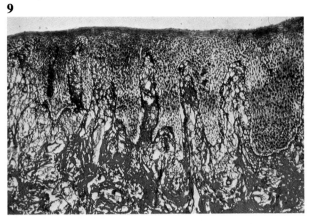

**9 Basement membrane.** Using a silver impregnation technique, the 'basement membrane' is visualised as a black-stained line between the epithelium and the connective tissue. *(Robb–Smith)*

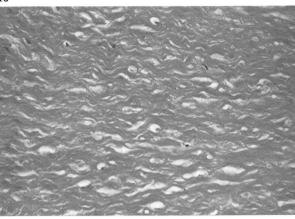

**10 Collagen fibres.** These stain red with the van Gieson's picro-fuchsin technique and form the principal extra-cellular element in the corium.

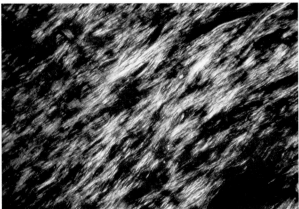

**11 Collagen fibres (polarised light).** Under polarised light, collagen fibres are visualised as bright white fibres in a black background. They exhibit the property of birefringence or 'double refraction'.

**12 Artery.** The artery has three recognisable layers, tunica intima, tunica media and tunica adventitia. The smooth muscle layer is well developed in the tunica media.

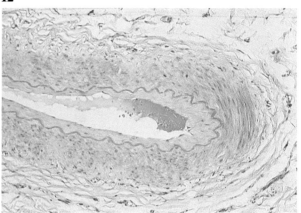

**13 Arteriole and vein.** These vessels have thinner muscular coats than the arteries with the vein being even more thin-walled than the arteriole.

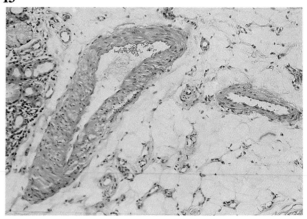

**14 Capillaries.** These are plentiful in the corium of the oral mucosa. They are lined with a single layer of endothelial cells.

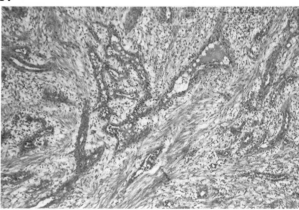

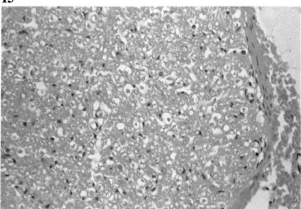

**15 Peripheral nerves.** In transverse section these appear as hollow tubes with a central axis cylinder and are surrounded by an endoneurium, perineurium and epineurium from within outwards.

**16 Collagen fibre bundles and peripheral nerve.** The similarities and differences between the two can be seen here. Both exhibit the 'snake fence' appearance, but the peripheral nerve below is distinctly more basophilic.

**17 Fordyce spots.** These are ectopic sebaceous glands beneath the buccal mucosa and appear clinically as buff-coloured granules.

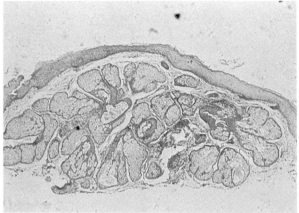

**18 Hypertrophy of foliate papillae.** Occasionally, patients complain of swellings on the lateral border of the tongue. These patients are often cancerophobic. Excision of the swellings show them to be foliate papillae of normal appearance.

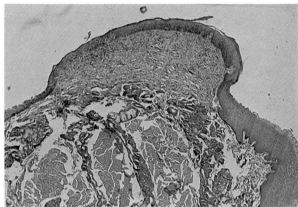

**19**

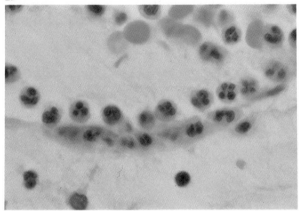

**20**

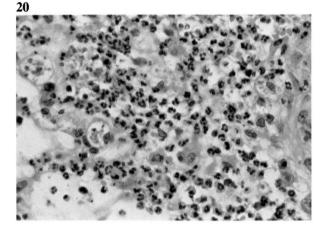

**19 Polymorphonuclear leucocytes** or neutrophil leucocytes are recognised by their multilobed nuclei and slightly basophilic granular cytoplasm.

**20 Polymorphonuclear leucocytes.** The appearance of these in large numbers in the extravascular tissues usually signifies an acute inflammatory cell reaction.

**21 Eosinophil leucocytes.** Like polymorphonuclear leucocytes, these are granular leucocytes and their eosinophilic granular cytoplasm can be seen to advantage in this special stain. *(Azoeosin)*

**21**

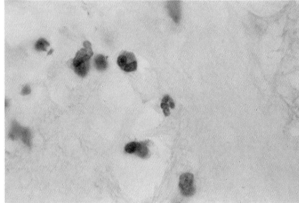

**22 Lymphocytes and plasma cells.** These inflammatory cells are commonly seen in chronic inflammation. Lymphocytes are small round cells which are almost all nucleus with very little recognisable cytoplasm. They are the most important cells of the immune system and increasingly sophisticated immunocytochemical techniques are being developed to aid their precise identification. Plasma cells seen on the right are larger cells with eccentric nuclei and a basophilic cytoplasm. Unless visualised under very high magnification, the cart-wheel appearance of the nucleus is not usually seen. The juxtanuclear halo is present in cells cut in a favourable plane.

**22**

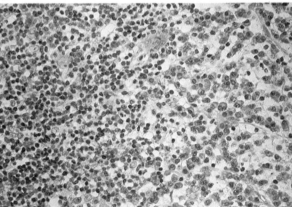

**23**

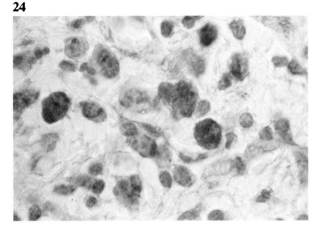

**24**

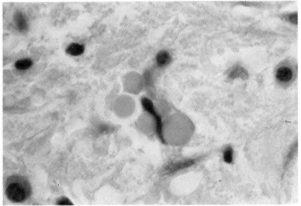

**23 Plasma cells.** These are rich in ribonucleic acid in their cytoplasm, as they are antibody-producing cells. The ribonucleic acid content can be demonstrated by the methyl-green pyronin method shown here, and the juxta-nuclear haloes are also evident.

**24 Plasma cells.** A particular class of immuno-globin produced by the plasma cell can be demonstrated as a brown reaction product with the immuno-peroxidase method. The particular immunoglobulin in this case is IgG.

**25 Russell bodies.** These appear as rounded eosinophilic bodies which are larger than red blood cells and do not have nuclei. They are thought to be aggregations of immunoglobulin produced by plasma cells.

**25**

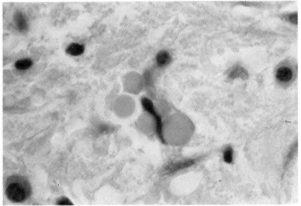

**26**

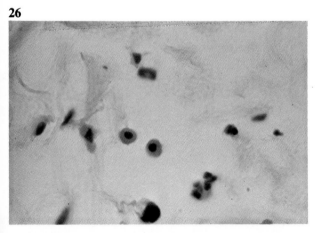

**27**

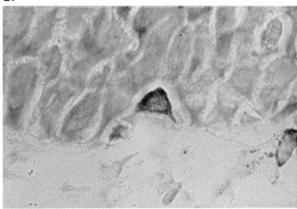

**26 Mast cells.** In haematoxylin-eosin stained paraffin sections these cells are not easily recognised. In its more characteristic form, the mast cell is a fairly large ovoid cell with a central, dark-staining nucleus and eosinophilic granular cytoplasm.

**27 Mast cells.** In toluidine blue-stained preparations, mast cells exhibit metachromasia. The cytoplasmic granules stain a purplish colour in contrast to the other cells which stain the colour of the dye.

**28 Histiocytes or macrophages** are not recognised easily by their morphology in routine histological preparations. They are usually identified on evidence of phagocytosed material. In this section the cells have engulfed a lipid material and appear as 'foam cells'.

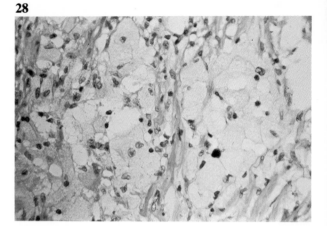

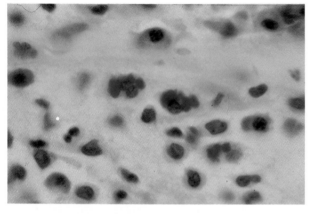

**29 Histiocytes containing haemosiderin.** The histiocytes have engulfed haemosiderin granules which are breakdown products of haemoglobin.

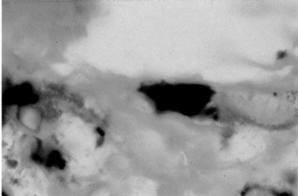

**30 Histiocytes containing haemosiderin.** The haemosiderin granules in histiocytes can be demonstrated by Perl's Prussian-blue reaction as a blue reaction product.

**31 Melanophages.** These are macrophages which have engulfed melanin.

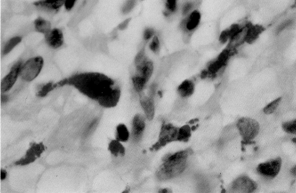

# (ii) Histological changes of importance in mucosal epithelium

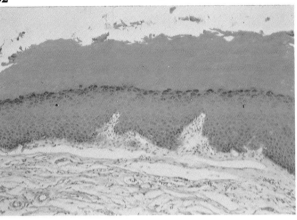

**32**

**32 Orthokeratosis/Hyperorthokeratosis.** This change describes the presence of a keratin layer on the surface of stratified squamous epithelium. The keratin layer does not contain cell nuclei and may exhibit a basket-weave pattern. A well-formed stratum granulosum is usually present.

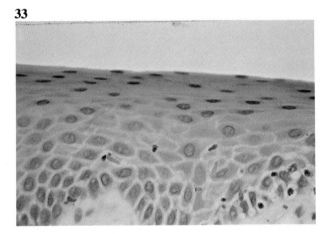

**33**

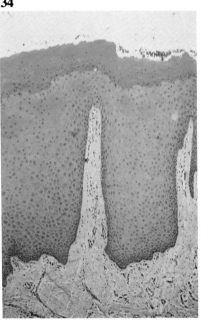

**34**

**33 Parakeratosis.** This change also describes the presence of a keratin layer but the persistence of nuclei distinguishes it from orthokeratosis and a well-formed stratum granulosum is not present, although occasional granular cells may be seen. Parakeratosis may occur as a normal variant of keratinization in the mouth, particularly on the gingiva.

**34 Acanthosis.** The epithelial layer is thickened with the formation of long and broad rete processes as a result of hyperplasia of the prickle-cell layer.

**35 Atrophy.** The epithelial layer is thinned with the reduction of thickness affecting chiefly the prickle-cell layer.

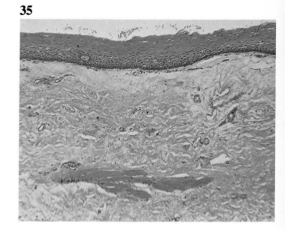

**36 Ulceration.** The covering epithelium has been destroyed, exposing the connective tissue. A small edge of normal epithelium is still visible. A thick layer of fibrin threads and polymorpho-nuclear leucocytes covers the surface of the corium.

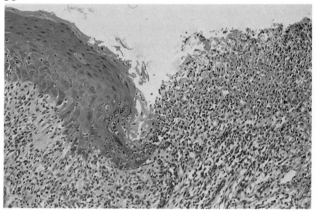

**37 Spongiosis (intercellular oedema).** The accumulation of intercellular fluid between the cells of the prickle-cell layer results in the separation of the cells from one another. The intercellular bridges, however, remain distinct.

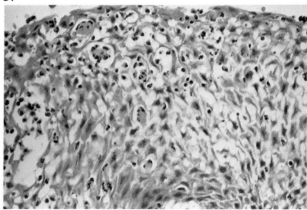

**38 Intra-epithelial vesicle/bulla formation.** A blister has formed within the layers of the epithelium. Both roof and floor of the vesicle are composed of epithelium.

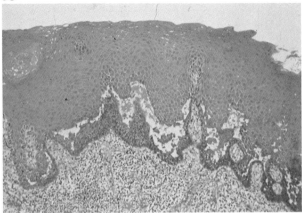

**39 Subepithelial bulla formation.** A blister has formed between epithelium and connective tissue. The floor consists of the corium.

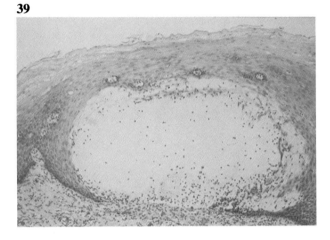

**40 Intracellular oedema.** Accumulation of fluid has taken place within the cytoplasm of the cells giving them a vacuolated appearance.

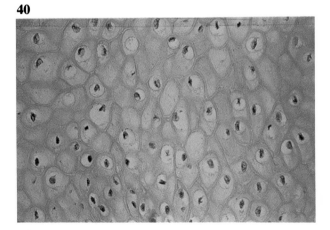

**41 Individual cell keratinization.** Keratin formation has taken place within the cytoplasm of the prickle-cells deep within the epithelium.

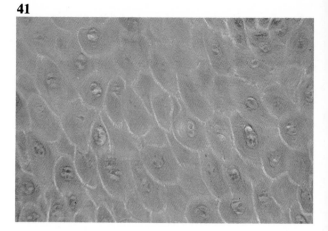

**42 Pseudoepitheliomatous hyperplasia.** An appearance which mimics an invasive carcinoma histologically, but is benign biologically, although its distinction from carcinoma can be difficult. Sometimes it is secondary to another condition which, if recognised, resolves the problem. (See page 103 .)

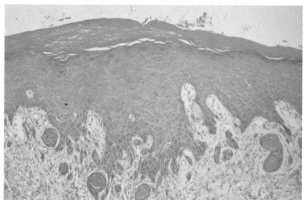

**43 Microabscess formation.** A small abscess may form within the epithelium with diffuse accumulation of polymorphonuclear leucocytes.

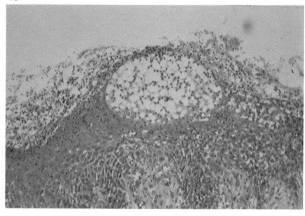

**44**

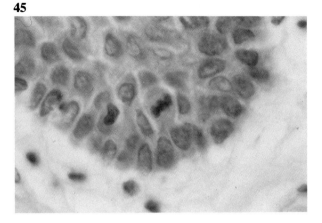

**45**

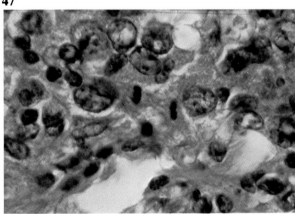

**44 Mitotic figure.** Prophase. It is extremely difficult to locate at light microscopic level a cell in early prophase. The cell shown here is probably in late prophase–early metaphase. The nuclear membrane is no longer distinct and condensation of chromatin is already evident.

**45 Mitotic figure.** Metaphase. Condensation of chromatin around the equatorial plate results in the formation of a 'bow-tie' figure.

**46 Mitotic figure.** Anaphase. Separation of the two 'daughter' nuclei is starting to take place.

**46**

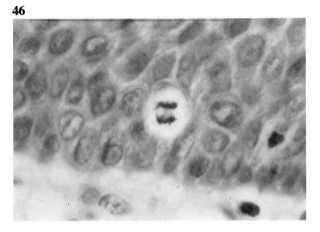

**47 Mitotic figure.** Telophase. Constriction of the cytoplasm results in the formation of two separate cells.

**47**

# (iii) White, ulcerative and bullous lesions

## Leukoplakia

This term is defined as '*a white patch on the oral mucosa which is not less than 5mm in diameter and which cannot be attributed to any known disease*'. Accordingly, the histology of such lesions is variable and ranges from the appearance of a keratin layer on a normally non-keratinized epithelium or an increase of thickness of a previously existing keratinized layer to severe changes throughout the epithelium. Only the milder changes are shown in this section. Other findings are shown in Chapter 6.

**48**

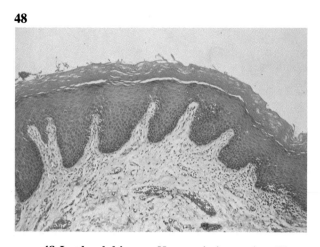

**48 Leukoplakia** – Hyperorthokeratosis. The keratin layer is thickened but the other layers of the epithelium appear normal.

**49**

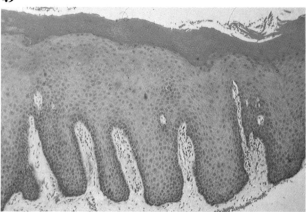

**49 Leukoplakia** – Parakeratosis and acanthosis. The covering epithelium exhibits orthokeratosis or parakeratosis and acanthosis. The rete processes are long and broad.

**50 Leukoedema.** The epithelium appears to be vacuolated throughout the greater part of its thickness. Most authorities now regard it as a variant of the normal buccal mucosa.

**50**

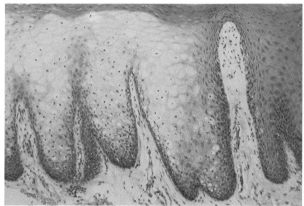

**51**

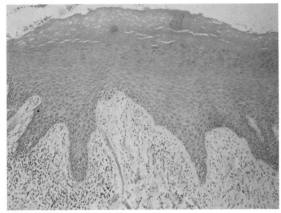

**52**

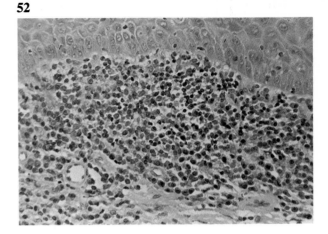

**51 Lichen planus.** The oral lesions of lichen planus are similar in appearance histologically to those of the skin, with minor modifications. In a low power view, the covering epithelium is ortho- or parakeratinized. The epithelial–connective tissue junction is irregular, but a 'saw-tooth' appearance is usually not attained. Civatte bodies and liquefaction degeneration of the basal layer of the epithelium are seen. There is a predominantly lymphocytic infiltrate close to the epithelial–connective tissue junction.

**52 Lichen planus.** Higher power view showing the band-like inflammatory cell infiltrate consisting mainly of lymphocytes at the epithelial–connective tissue junction.

**53**

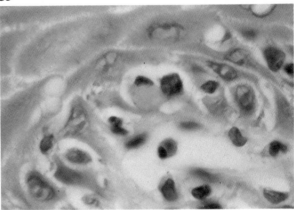

**53 Civatte bodies.** Civatte or Colloid bodies appear as eosinophilic rounded masses in the basal cell layer with darkly stained basophilic nuclear fragments. They are thought to represent a type of degeneration involving epithelial cells usually referred to as programmed cell death.

**54 Liquefaction degeneration.** At the level of the light microscope, this is thought to represent a degenerative change affecting the basal cell layer of the epithelium and an eosinophilic zone replaces part or all of the basal cell layer.

**54**

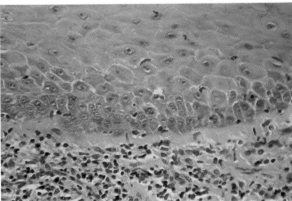

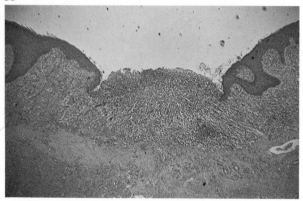

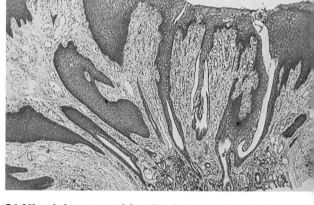

**55 Histologically non-specific oral ulcer.** The covering stratified squamous epithelium is breached, the underlying corium exposed and the surface covered with a film of fibrin and polymorphonuclear leucocytes. A diffuse chronic inflammatory cell infiltrate is seen at the base of the ulcer. This appearance is usual in any of the common forms of recurrent oral ulceration, such as minor and major aphthae, or traumatic ulcers.

**56 Nicotinic stomatitis** (Leukokeratosis nicotina palati). Clinically the palate appears white. Large papular swellings with small red spots at the centre are seen at the posterior part of the hard palate. Histologically the red spots represent the openings of mucous glands which are blocked by keratin plugs. The ducts leading from the mucous glands to the surface undergo squamous metaplasia.

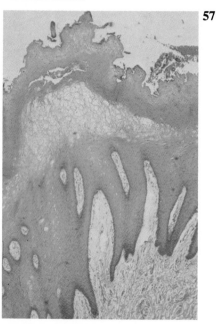

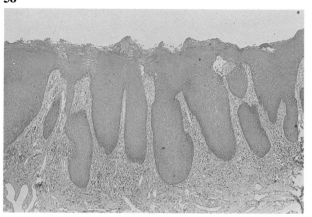

**57 White sponge naevus.** This is a developmental anomaly manifesting as white patches on the oral mucosa. It is inherited on an autosomal dominant basis and a family history is important in arriving at a diagnosis, as cheek biting (morsicatio buccarum) often gives rise to a similar clinical and histological appearance.

The covering stratified squamous epithelium is parakeratinized and exhibits acanthosis. The prickle-cell layer contains large numbers of vacuolated cells or cells with a 'washed out' appearance, and the underlying connective tissue is usually free from inflammatory cell infiltration. The surface of the epithelium is commonly covered with micro-organisms.

**58 Median rhomboid glossitis.** This was once regarded as a developmental anomaly due to persistence of the tuberculum impar. Considerable doubt has been thrown on this theory in recent years, however, as it is usually not seen in children.

The epithelium exhibits parakeratosis and acanthosis with 'test-tube' shaped rete processes. Candida hyphae and polymorphonuclear leucocyte infiltration are associated features, although Candida albicans as a primary cause of the condition remains unproven. A hyalinised band of fibrous tissue superficial to the tongue muscles is a constant finding, and this is thought to be part of the septum of the tongue.

**59 Erythema migrans (geographic tongue).** The histological features of this curious condition of unknown aetiology are very similar to a candidal infection but candida hyphae are not seen. The epithelium is poorly parakeratinized and markedly spongiotic with a diffuse polymorphonuclear leucocyte infiltration. The connective tissue is also diffusely infiltrated with inflammatory cells.

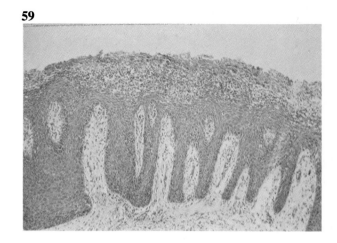

**60 Submucous fibrosis.** This 25-year-old Indian male complained of limitation of mouth opening. The pale fibrous bands of the buccal mucosa can be seen.

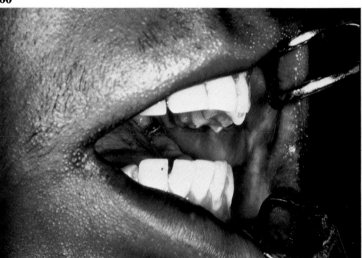

**61 Submucous fibrosis.** It is difficult, if not impossible, to make a histological diagnosis in the early stages, as the appearances are not specific. When advanced, however, the lamina propria is markedly collagenous and acellular, and the covering epithelium atrophic.

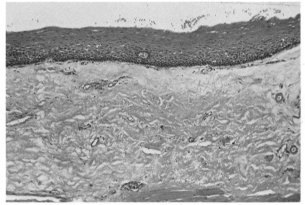

**62**

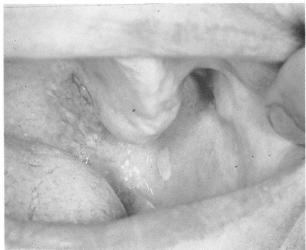

**62 Pemphigus vulgaris.** This 52-year-old female complained of oral ulceration for three months. A collapsed bulla can be seen on the buccal mucosa and erosive lesions are on the palate.

**63**

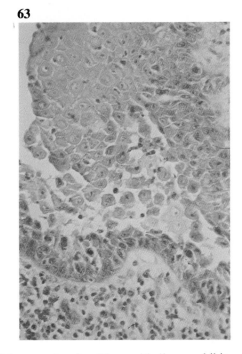

**63 Pemphigus vulgaris.** The epithelium exhibits supra-basal cleft formation and acantholytic or Tzanck cells are seen within the intra-epithelial bulla.

**64**

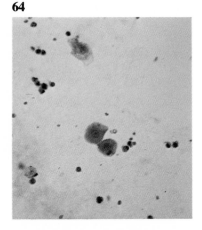

**64 Acantholytic cells in cytological smears.** Cytological smears from intact or recently ruptured bullae often provide useful confirmatory diagnostic features. Individual acantholytic cells are polyhedral with a centrally placed darkly staining nucleus and eosinophilic cytoplasm.

**65**

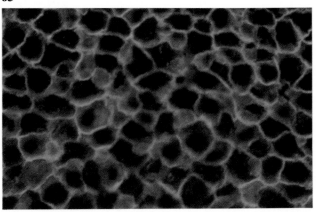

**65 Pemphigus vulgaris.** An indirect immunofluorescence photomicrograph shows the presence of antibodies to intercellular substance in the prickle-cell layer of mucosal epithelium.

**66 Benign mucous membrane pemphigoid.** This condition usually affects elderly females and not uncommonly presents as chronic desquamative gingivitis, as in this 62-year-old woman.

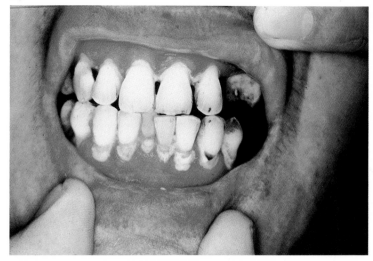

**67 Benign mucous membrane pemphigoid.** An unruptured bulla can be seen on the gingiva above ⁄6.

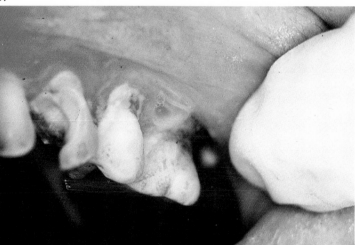

**68 Benign mucous membrane pemphigoid.** In contrast to true pemphigus, in this condition the bullae are sub-epithelial. The whole thickness of the epithelium forms the roof and the corium the floor.

**69 Benign mucous membrane pemphigoid.** Indirect immunofluorescence reveals the presence of antibodies to the basement membrane region.

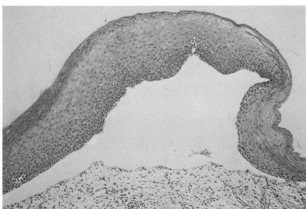

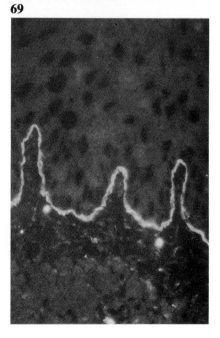

# 2 Non-neoplastic soft tissue swellings

**70 Fibroepithelial hyperplasia.** This is the most common lump in the oral mucosa. The lesional tissue is usually mature collagenous fibrous tissue often arranged in criss-cross bundles and with a varying amount of inflammatory cell infiltration. The covering epithelium may be keratinized as a result of friction.

**70**

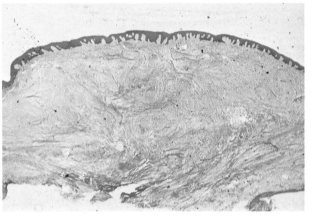

**71 'Giant cell fibroma'.** In this form of hyperplasia the surface is often papillomatous. The fibroblasts exhibit a variation in morphology with angular, stellate and multinucleate forms in addition to the more usual spindle-shaped cells.

**71**

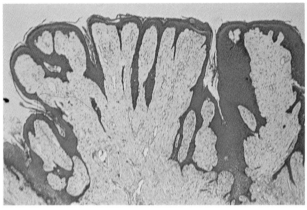

**72 'Giant cell fibroma'.** The variation in cytology with the formation of angular, stellate-shaped, and binucleated or multinucleated cells is shown in this higher power view.

**72**

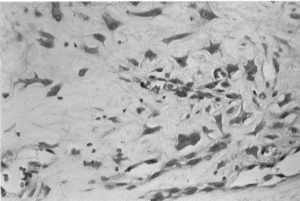

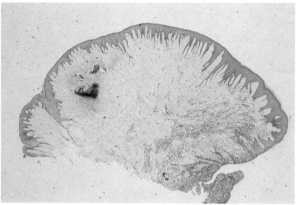

**73 Fibrous epulis.** This is a term restricted to a form of fibro-epithelial hyperplasia occurring on the gingiva. It is fairly collagenous and covered with a keratinized or parakeratinized stratified squamous epithelium. Metaplastic bone may form in a fibrous epulis.

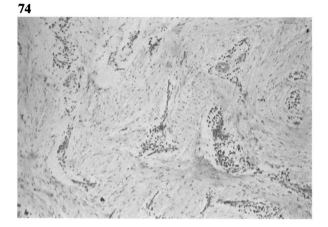

**74 Fibrous epulis.** Focal aggregations of chronic inflammatory cells are often seen around small blood vessels.

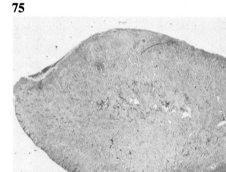

**75 Calcifying fibroblastic granuloma** (peripheral fibroma with calcification, peripheral ossifying fibroma). This is a variant of the fibrous epulis with a characteristic clinical and histological appearance. It usually affects individuals in the second decade and tends to recur. Cellular fibroblastic connective tissue forms the principal component and multiple foci of acellular calcifications are frequently present. The surface is usually ulcerated.

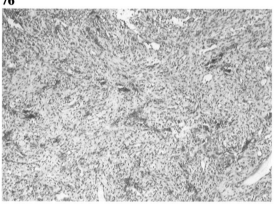

**76 Calcifying fibroblastic granuloma.** Higher power view showing the cellular fibroblastic connective tissue and the foci of calcification and ossification.

**77 Pyogenic granuloma.** The surface is extensively ulcerated and vasoformative tissue forms the chief component of the lesion. The degree of vascularity is so pronounced that it is difficult, if not impossible, to differentiate between it and a capillary haemangioma.

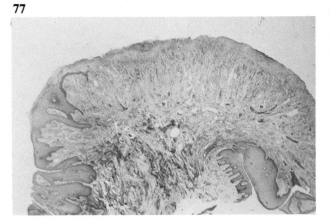

**78 Pyogenic granuloma.** Note the dilated capillaries lined with endothelial cells in a delicate fibrous connective tissue stroma. Similar lesions in pregnant women are referred to as 'pregnancy epulides'.

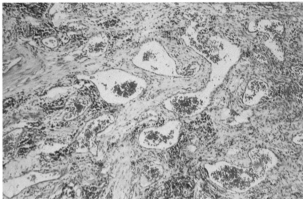

**79 Pyogenic granuloma.** Sometimes the vasoformative response is seen as areas of solid endothelial proliferation with incipient canalisation of the small vessels.

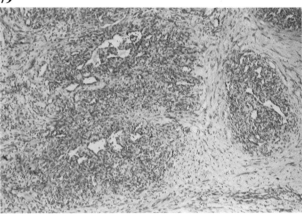

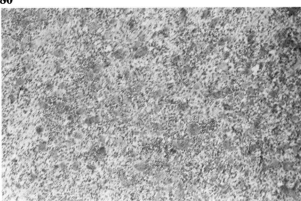

**80 Giant cell epulis – vascular confluent type** (peripheral giant cell granuloma). Multinucleated giant cells in a mononuclear cell stroma are often seen with foci of haemorrhage. More collagenous fibrous tissue separates the foci of giant cells. This lesion should not be confused with the 'giant cell fibroma'.

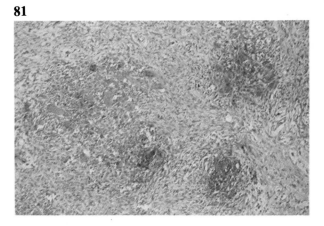

**81 Giant cell epulis – spindle cell type.** Two variants of the giant cell epulis are recognised. In the vascular confluent variety, the giant cells are not easily separated from the mononuclear 'stromal' cells. In the spindle cell variety shown here, they are more distinct.

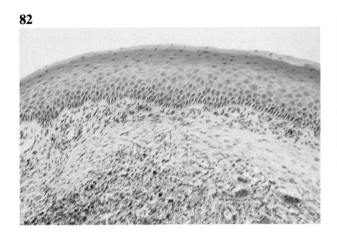

**82 Giant cell epulis.** The lesional tissue in a giant cell epulis is normally separated from the overlying epithelium by a band of normal corium. Histiocytes containing haemosiderin are usually prominent in this zone.

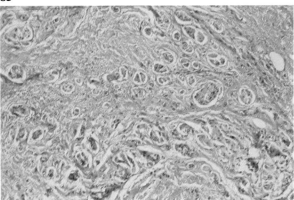

**83 Traumatic or amputation neuroma.** This lesion manifests as a painful swelling resulting from trauma to the peripheral nerve. When a peripheral nerve is severed and regeneration from the proximal end is overexuberant, a mass of distorted nerve fibres is seen.

**84 Idiopathic gingivofibromatosis.** The histological appearances in this condition are not different from normal gingivae. The corium may be indistinguishable from normal gingivae or may be more collagenous. Inflammatory cell infiltrate, if present, is usually mild and the covering keratinized epithelium is normal.

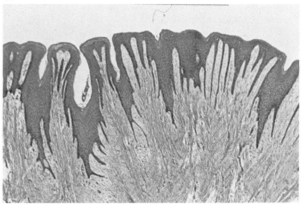

**85 Phenytoin hyperplasia** (Epanutin or dilantin hyperplasia). The covering epithelium is hyperplastic with long thin rete processes. Radiating bundles of collagen are seen and inflammatory cell infiltration is usually absent or mild.

**86 Papillary hyperplasia of the palate.** The irregular surface reflects the clinical picture. Marked acanthosis resulting in pseudo-epitheliomatous hyperplasia is often an associated feature. The connective tissue is usually diffusely infiltrated with inflammatory cells.

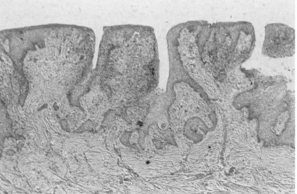

**87 Verruciform xanthoma.** This is a lesion of unknown aetiology, but presents with a clinical appearance similar to some fibroepithelial hyperplasias. The surface is papillomatous, and the epithelium exhibits hyperparakeratosis.

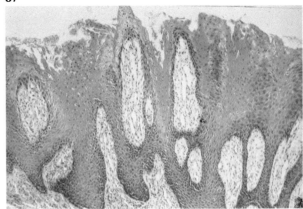

**88 Verruciform xanthoma.** Higher power examination shows the presence of many foam cells within the dermal papillae.

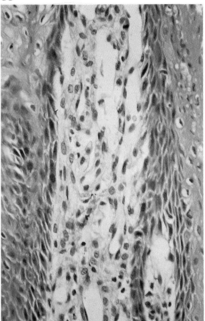

**89 Denture granuloma (denture hyperplasia).** This is a form of inflammatory hyperplasia related to the edges of ill-fitting dentures. The histology is similar to other types of inflammatory hyperplasia, except that the groove in which the denture edge rests is often ulcerated, as shown here, and some of them may be secondarily infected by Candida albicans.

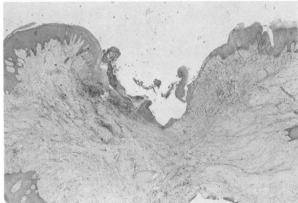

# 3 Disorders of bone

**90**

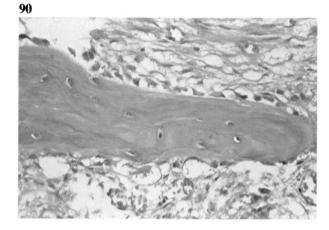

**90 Osteoblasts or bone forming cells.** These are recognised as a row of polyhedral cells on the surface of the bone.

**91**

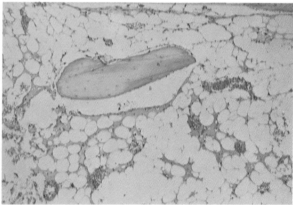

**91 Osteoclasts.** These are multinucleated giant cells resting in resorption bays, called Howship's lacunae, on the surface of the bone that is being resorbed.

**92**

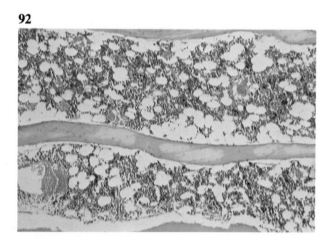

**92 Haemopoietic marrow in cancellous bone.** Higher power view showing the forming blood cells in cancellous bone containing haemopoietic marrow. Certain sites in the jaw bones, such as the mandibular condyle and the third molar region, retain haemopoietic marrow until an advanced age. This appearance must not be confused with inflammation of the marrow spaces.

**93**

**93 Fatty marrow.** Adipose tissue is found in other parts of the jaws within normal adult marrow spaces.

**94**

![woven bone formation micrograph]

**95**

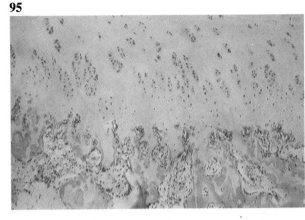

**94 Woven bone formation.** In the adult this bone is formed in the initial stages of repair. The trabeculae are slender and the collagen fibres do not show a lamellated appearance. It is also called coarse-fibred woven bone and fibrous tissue replaces the marrow between the bony trabeculae.

**95 Endochondral ossification.** This is the normal mode of bone formation in long bones where a pre-formed cartilage model is replaced by bone.

**96 Subperiosteal new bone deposition.** Subperiosteal bone deposition may occur as a response to disease. Both inflammatory and neoplastic conditions may stimulate the formation of new bone. Here parallel trabeculae of new bone have been laid down. Radiologically this gives rise to an onion-peel effect.

**96**

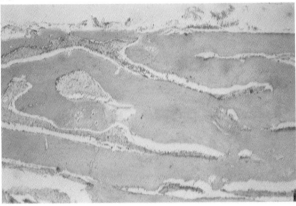

**97 Sclerosis of bone.** Enostosis appears radiographically as a radio-opaque mass within the bone and may be diagnosed as a cementoma. Histologically it can be seen to be composed of a dense mass of compact bone and may be regarded as a form of osteoma.

**97**

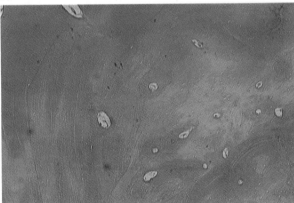

**98**

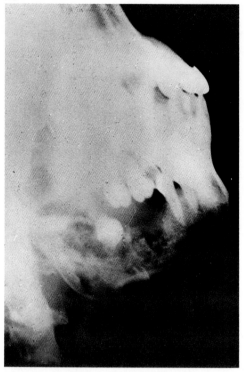

**99**

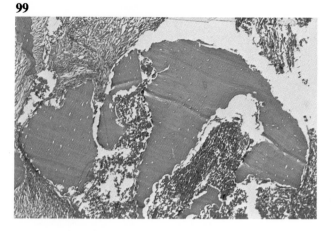

**99 Osteomyelitis.** As a result of inflammation of the soft tissues of the marrow, the bone undergoes necrosis; when the necrotic bone is separated from adjacent live bone it is called a sequestrum. The lacunae of the bone are empty and do not contain osteocytes. Granulation tissue and bacterial masses often cover the necrotic bone.

**98 Osteomyelitis.** Radiography shows the mottled appearance of the bone in an established case of osteomyelitis of the mandible.

**100**

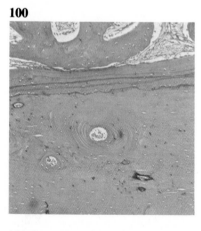

**100 Osteomyelitis.** Subperiosteal new bone formation on the surface of the cortex results in the formation of an involucrum.

**101**

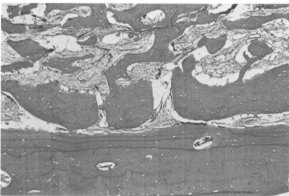

**101 Osteomyelitis.** Higher power view of the subperiosteal new bone that has formed on the surface of the cortex.

**102 Fibrous dysplasia.** Occlusal radiograph showing the ground glass appearance of the bone in a case of fibrous dysplasia of the mandible.

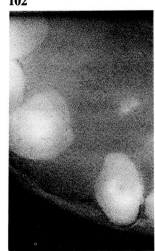

102

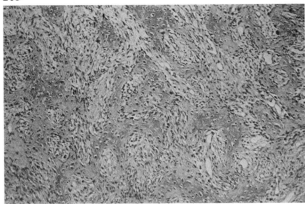

103

**103 Fibrous dysplasia.** Slender trabeculae of woven bone are seen in a cellular fibrous connective tissue stroma. The presence of osteoblasts is not commonly evident and the bone is considered metaplastic.

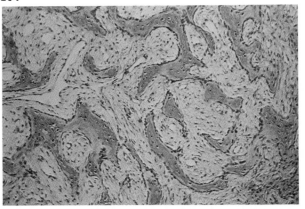

104

**104 Fibrous dysplasia.** In the jaw bones osteoblastic rimming of the bony trabeculae may be seen; this should not negate the diagnosis of fibrous dysplasia.

**105 Fibrous dysplasia.** When the lesion enters the inactive stage, the bony trabeculae may become lamellated, and both osteoblastic and osteoclastic activity ceases. Fibrous marrow is still evident.

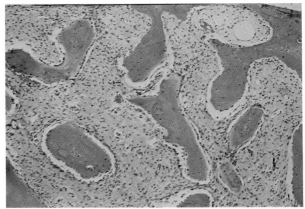

105

**106 Fibrous dysplasia.** An important distinction between fibrous dysplasia and ossifying fibroma is that the former merges into the normal bone while the latter is sharply demarcated and may possess a fibrous capsule. There may be fusion between the lesional tissue and cortical bone.

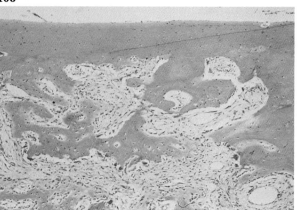

**107 Osteitis deformans (Paget's disease of bone).** In active Paget's disease there is marked osteoclastic and osteoblastic activity with fibrous replacement of the marrow. The marrow may be extremely vascular because of the presence of arteriovenous shunts.

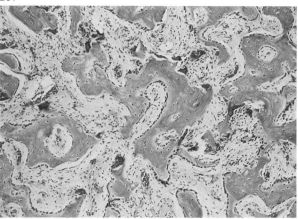

**108 Osteitis deformans (Paget's disease).** The result of the osteoclastic and osteoblastic activity is the formation of a mosaic pattern of the bone.

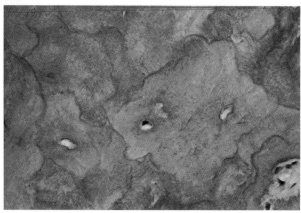

**109 'Brown node' of hyperparathy-roidism.** The 'brown-ness' of a giant cell granuloma is apparent. Since the clinical and histological features of giant cell granulomas and hyperparathyroidism are identical, blood chemistry studies must be undertaken to establish whether the serum calcium is elevated.

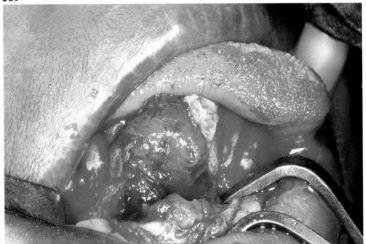

**110 Giant cell granuloma.** Central. Multi-nucleated giant cells are irregularly distributed in a haemorrhagic fibrous stroma.

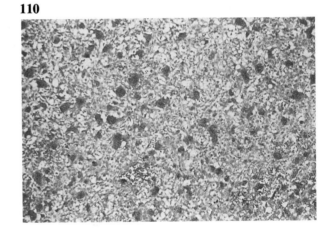

**111 Giant cell granuloma.** Central. Islands and trabeculae of bone and osteoid may form between the foci of giant cells.

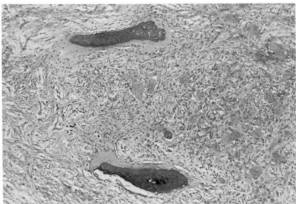

**112 Giant cell granuloma.** Central. Some examples of giant cell granuloma show the presence of islands of odontogenic epithelium. No differences in behaviour have been noted between those that have such islands and those that do not.

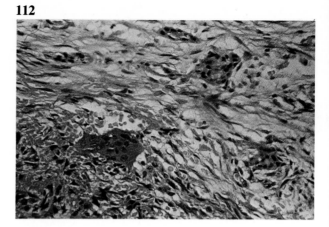

**113 Cherubism.** The histological features of cherubism are very similar to giant cell granulomas, although the clinical features and the pattern of genetic transmission make the diagnosis more obvious.

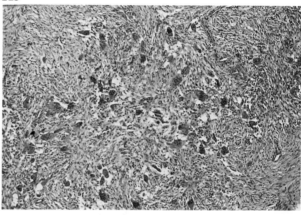

**114 Cherubism.** The hyalinised areas around blood vessels are said to be characteristic of the condition but are not seen in all cases. These areas are formed by hyalinised collagen bundles.

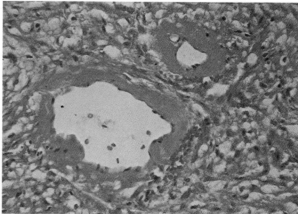

**115 Histiocytosis 'X'. Langerhans cell granulomatosis.** One of the manifestations of this curious disorder of unknown aetiology is the marked destruction of the periodontal tissues in young children.

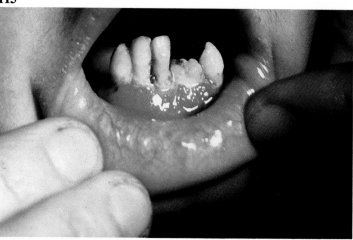

**116 Histiocytosis 'X'.** Radiography shows the marked destruction of the alveolar bone supporting the teeth.

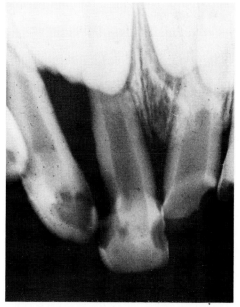

**117 Histiocytosis 'X'.** Histological features of the condition show that the predominant cells seen are histiocyte-like cells which are aggregated in sheets and eosinophil leucocytes. Ultrastructurally, these cells possess a characteristic cytoplasmic granule referred to as a Langerhans granule.

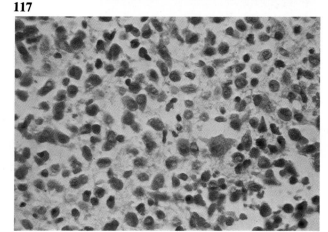

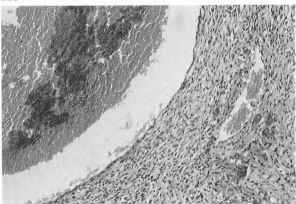

**118 Aneurysmal bone cyst.** Large vascular spaces lined with condensed fibroblasts form the cystic part of the lesion.

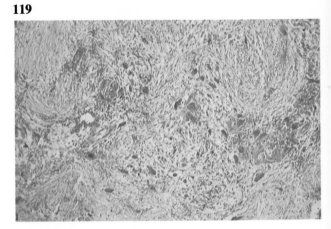

**119 Aneurysmal bone cyst.** The lesion may also contain many solid areas which are histologically indistinguishable from a giant cell granuloma.

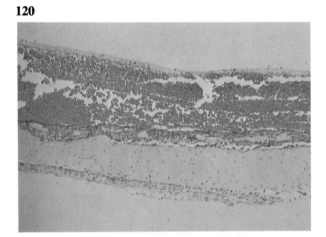

**120 Solitary bone cyst** (traumatic 'haemorrhagic' bone cyst). A thin bony plate lined with tenuous fibrous tissue is all that can be seen when the cystic cavity is explored. Sometimes a small amount of sero-sanguinous fluid is seen.

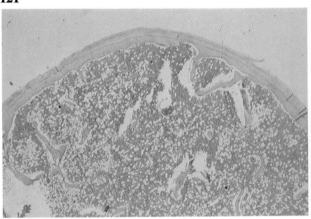

**121 Normal mandibular condyle.** Histology of a condyle removed from a 70-year-old man. Note the thin layer of fibro-cartilage covering the condyle and the underlying bone which still contains haemopoietic marrow.

**122**

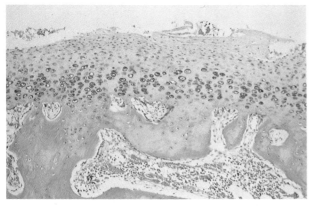

**122 Condylar hyperplasia.** This condyle was removed from a 25-year-old man who complained of increasing deviation of his jaws to one side. The fibro-cartilage layer is thickened showing that growth is still active.

**123**

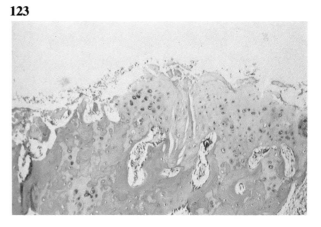

**123 Osteoarthrosis.** There is vertical splitting of the fibro-cartilage layer. Eventually this layer is completely lost, leaving the underlying bone exposed.

**124**

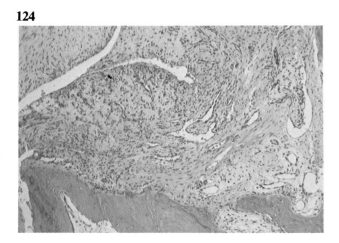

**124 Rheumatoid or infective arthritis.** The histology of a rheumatoid and an infective arthritis is very similar. Granulation tissue called pannus covers the exposed surfaces of the condyle which undergoes resorption.

**125**

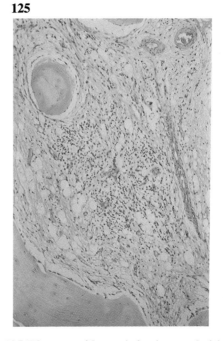

**125 Rheumatoid or infective arthritis.** The marrow spaces are replaced by fibrous tissue and chronic inflammatory cell infiltration is seen.

# 4 Pathology of dental and periodontal tissues

## (i) Dental caries and its sequelae
## Caries of enamel

Smooth surface lesions

**126 Early enamel caries** – transmitted light. The early carious lesion on a smooth surface is cone-shaped, with the tip pointing towards the dentine. The dark zone is clearly seen but the other zones are not evident.

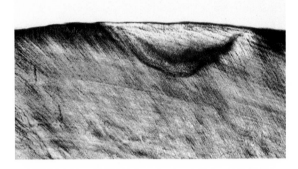

**127 Early enamel caries** – polarised light and first order red plate. The use of polarised light and a retardation plate results in the production of interference colours, and the dark zone exhibits positive birefringence in contrast to the rest of the lesion. (*Synthetic mount R1 1.524*)

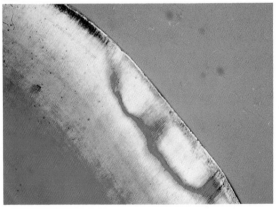

**128 Early enamel caries** – polarised light and first order red plate. The 'body' of the lesion is seen to be 'bi-lobed' in this case and the striae of Retzius are enhanced within the carious lesion. The surface zone is negatively birefringent, and the dark zone is enveloped by the body of the lesion. (*Water mount RI 1.33*)

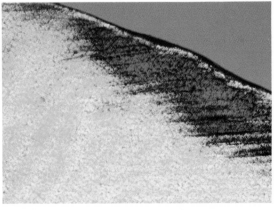

**129**

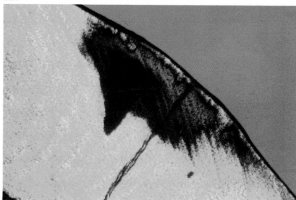

**130**

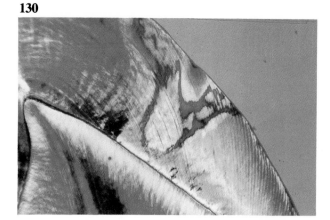

**129 More advanced enamel caries** – polarised light and first order red plate. The cone-shaped lesion has extended further and the striae of Retzius appear to provide the natural pathways of spread. More recent scanning electron microscopic studies suggest that the reverse is the case, i.e. the striae actually offer increased resistance to caries attack. *(Water mount RI 1.33)*

**130 Late enamel caries** – polarised light and first order red plate. The dark zone has almost reached the amelo-dentinal junction and a second dark zone has formed within the body of the lesion. The surface zone has been breached. *(Synthetic mount RI 1.524)*

Fissure caries

**131**

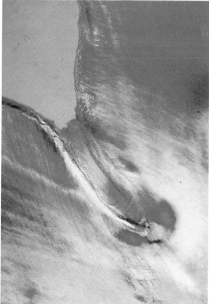

**132**

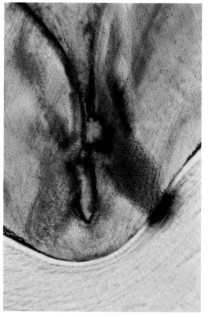

**131 Occlusal caries** – polarised light and first order red plate. Two small zones of positive birefringence have formed on both side walls of the central fissure. *(Synthetic mount RI 1.524)*

**132 Occlusal caries.** The carious lesion in the depths of an occlusal fissure is dependent upon the shape of the fissure. In narrow fissures the lesion commences on one or both of the side walls and spreads outwards towards the amelo-dentinal junction resulting in the formation of a conical lesion, with the tip of the cone pointing towards the surface. In this case only one of the walls of the fissure has been affected, and the caries has spread to the dentine.

**141**

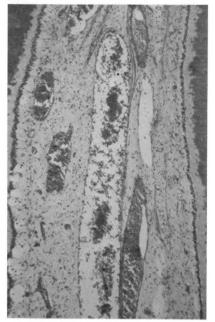

**141 Hyperaemia.** The blood vessels engorged with blood cells can be seen in parts of the pulp that are free from inflammatory cell infiltration.

**142**

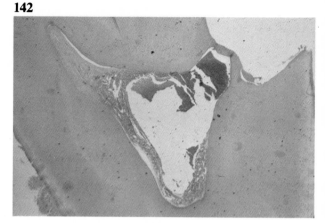

**142 Pulp abscess.** The pulp chamber is occupied by an abscess cavity which appears to be largely empty because the lipid material has been dissolved out during preparation of the section.

**143**

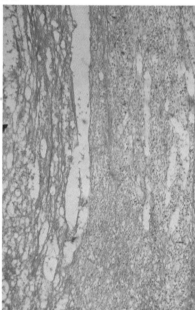

**143 Necrosis of the pulp.** All structural details are now lost; nuclei of any remaining cells exhibit pyknosis, karyolysis and karyorrhexis.

**144**

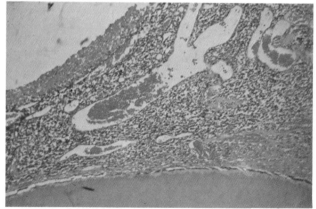

**144 Part of the wall of the abscess.** The wall of the abscess is formed by granulation tissue diffusely infiltrated by both polymorphonuclear leucocytes and chronic inflammatory cells. Within the abscess cavity are dead or dying polymorphonuclear leucocytes, so-called 'pus-cells'.

**145 Chronic open pulpitis** (chronic 'ulcerative' pulpitis). The pulp is widely exposed, and the pulp chamber filled with granulation tissue which has replaced the normal pulp tissue. There is diffuse infiltration by inflammatory cells.

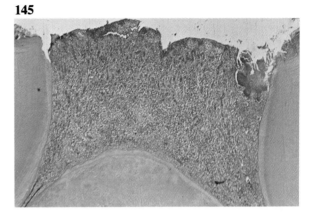

**146 Chronic hyperplastic pulpitis** – pulp polypus. This is similar to chronic 'ulcerative' pulpitis. The granulation tissue has mushroomed out of the pulp chamber and fills a large part of the carious cavity.

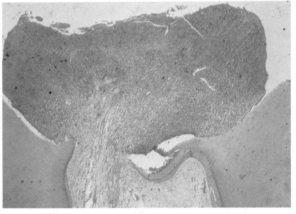

**147 Chronic hyperplastic pulpitis.** After it has been exposed to the oral cavity, the pulp polypus acquires a covering of stratified squamous epithelium. This is the result of shed epithelial cells having been seeded on the surface of the granulation tissue, and forming a 'graft'.

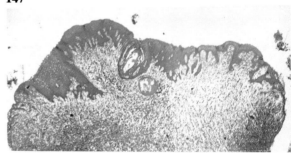

**148**

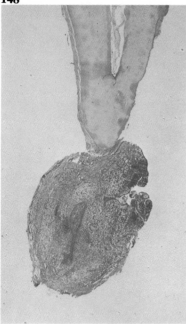

**149**

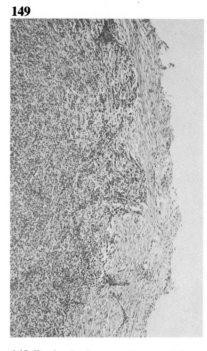

**148 Periapical granuloma.** This is a mass of granulation tissue that has formed around the apex of a tooth that has succumbed to caries. It contains proliferating epithelium and is diffusely infiltrated with inflammatory cells. More collagenous fibrous tissue is seen at the periphery, forming a capsule.

**149 Periapical granuloma.** More collagenous fibrous tissue forms a capsule around the granulation tissue.

**150**

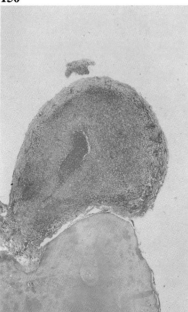

**151**

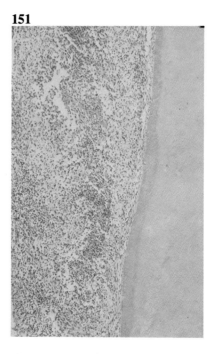

**150 Periapical granuloma.** Breakdown of the periapical granuloma to an abscess occurs often and the cellular composition of the granulation tissue mass is variable.

**151 Acute periodontitis.** This section was prepared from a tooth which was tender to percussion. A diffuse predominantly polymorphonuclear leucocyte infiltrate is seen in the periodontal ligament. The pulp was necrotic.

# (ii) Reactions to operative procedures and trauma

**152**

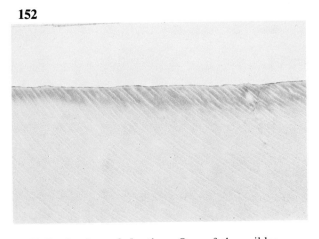

**152 Darkening of dentine.** One of the milder effects of cavity preparation with high speed instrumentation is the darkening of dentine. The surface zone of the dentine at the floor of the cavity is more deeply staining than the rest of the dentine.

**153**

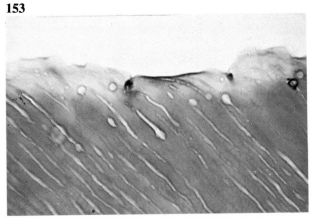

**153 Burning of dentine.** This is a more severe change affecting the dentine. The surface of the dentine is less heavily stained and it has often a pleated appearance. The affected tubules may show dilatation and a beaded appearance.

**154**

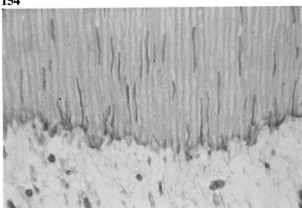

**154 Aspiration of odontoblasts.** This is a phenomenon which is observed immediately postoperatively; nuclei of odontoblasts have been aspirated into the tubules as a result of dehydration of the surface of the cavity with resultant fluid movement from the pulp.

**155**

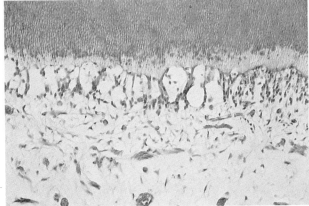

**155 Fluid disturbance.** Vacuoles or 'blisters' may form in the odontoblast layer, and with some filling materials a large area of the pulp may be involved. Because this change may sometimes be artefactual, it is important to accept only those vacuoles which are limited to the actual area of operation as genuine.

**156**

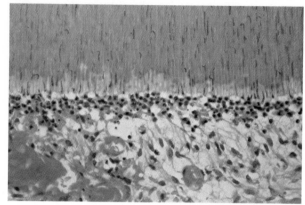

**156 Inflammatory cell infiltration – polymorphonuclear leucocytes.** This is usually seen in the region of the odontoblast layer about 24 hours postoperatively.

**157**

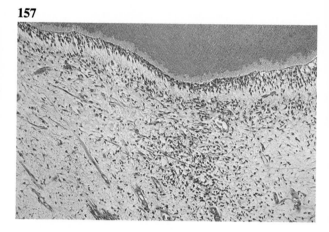

**157 Inflammatory cell infiltration – chronic inflammatory cells.** This is usually seen 48 to 72 hours later, as a focus of lymphocytes, plasma cells and macrophages, in the deeper part of the pulp.

**158**

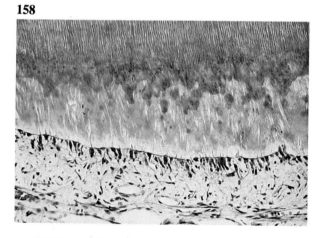

**158 Reparative dentine formation.** This is not usually observed earlier than 14 days postoperatively. After that it shows a gradual increase in dentine formation for several months.

**159**

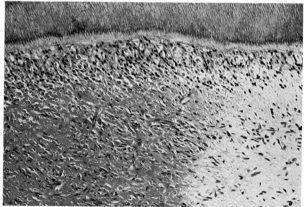

**159 Coagulative necrosis.** High speed instrumentation in cavity preparation without an adequate coolant results in severe changes like this affecting the pulp.

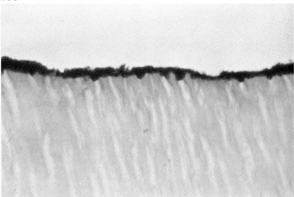

**160**

**160 Alteration in staining of cavity wall in contact with self-curing acrylic resins.** Some self-curing acrylic resins employ a sealing agent to effect a better union between filling material and cavity wall. This particular material contained glycerophosphoric acid dimethacrylate to effect such a bond.

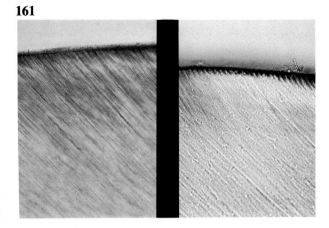

**161**

**161 Acid-etched enamel surface.** In this split photomicrograph, the right side had been etched with 50% orthophosphoric acid for 1 minute, while the left side shows normal enamel. Small wedge-shaped defects can be seen on the surface of the etched enamel, and these allow 'tags' to be formed with the composite resin used to restore the tooth.

**162**

**162 Amalgam tattoo.** These appear as pigmented lesions in the oral mucosa and may be confused with melanotic lesions. Particles of dental amalgam have been impregnated in the lamina propria and have provoked a foreign body reaction.

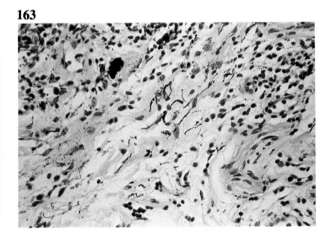

**163**

**163 Amalgam tattoo.** Sometimes the collagen fibres may be impregnated with the corrosion products of dental amalgam.

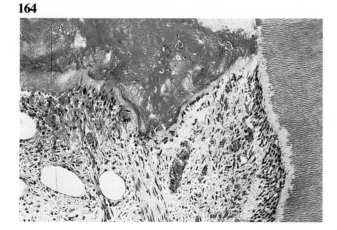

**164 Pulp capping.** If the procedure of pulp capping is successful, a dentine bridge is formed, as shown.

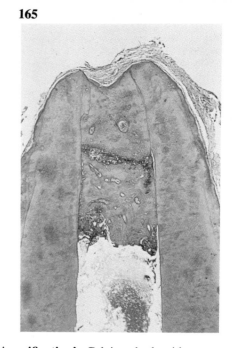

**165 'Apexification'.** Calcium hydroxide preparations are used also to treat teeth with open apices to stimulate closure of the apex. If the procedure is successful, a perfect apical seal can be obtained.

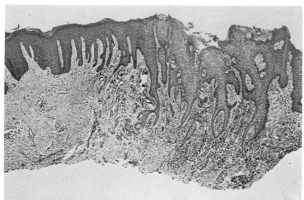

**166 Effects of restorations on the gingiva.** This biopsy is taken from the subpontic area of a fixed bridge. The covering epithelium is markedly acanthotic and there is a diffuse inflammatory cell infiltrate in the lamina propria.

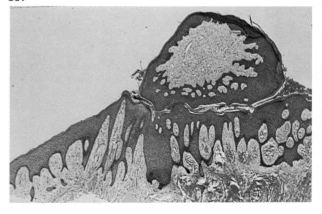

**167 Epulis formation.** Prolonged irritation, whether mechanical or bacterial, beneath the subpontic area may result in the formation of an epulis.

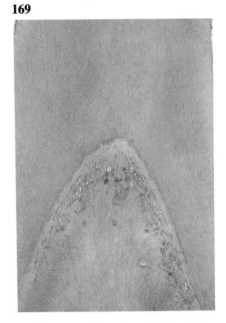

**168 Reaction to trauma.** An additional cusp appears to have developed at the dilaceration.

**169 Reaction to trauma.** A marked calcio-traumatic line marks the episode of trauma, and the dentine that forms after the episode may be completely atubular or cellular.

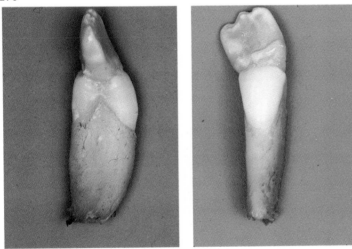

**170 Reaction to trauma.** This tooth was subjected to trauma during an early stage of its development. The crown is dilacerated and hypoplastic but the tooth went on to full root formation.

**171 Reaction to trauma.** If the odontoblasts survive after the accident, little or no difference may be noticed between the dentine that is formed after the episode. *(Picrothionin)*

**172**

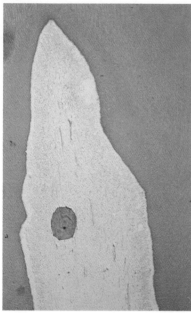

**172 Aseptic necrosis of the pulp.** If the pulp succumbs following the trauma, aseptic necrosis of the pulp may result. Little cellular detail is seen, but the structural integrity of the architecture is retained.

**173**

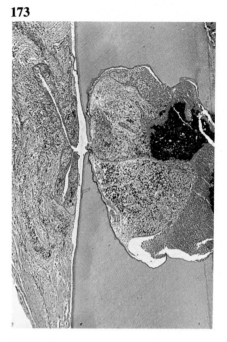

**173 Perforation of the lateral aspect of the root.** Accidental perforation of the root may take place during root canal therapy. Granulation tissue has filled the defect and histiocytes have engulfed part of the root filling material.

**174**

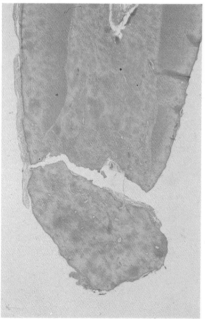

**174 Reaction to trauma.** The pulp may be entirely obliterated following trauma. In this case, a root fracture has developed additionally.

**175**

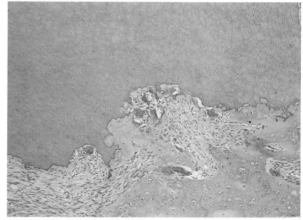

**175 Resorption of dental tissues.** All three calcified dental tissues may be resorbed by osteoclast-like cells. The enamel of buried teeth, dentine and cementum may be affected under a wide variety of circumstances. Resorption of dentine may take place internally, resulting in the formation of a pink-spot clinically.

**176**

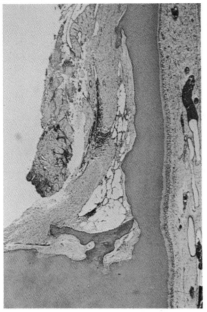

**177**

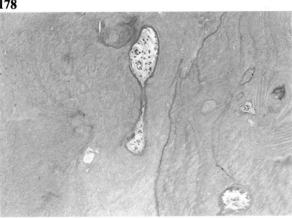

**177 Burrowing external resorption.** Resorption is accompanied by repair; a bone-like calcific tissue of repair may replace the resorbed dentine.

**176 Burrowing external resorption.** This commences beneath the gingival crevice and burrows its way under the crown, also presenting as a pink-spot clinically. A narrow zone of dentine separates the resorbed area from the pulp which remains vital and normal until the resorptive process reaches it.

**179**

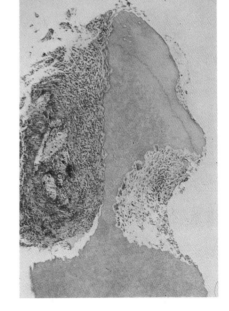

**178**

**178 Ankylosis.** The alternate resorption and repair of dental tissues may result in ankylosis of the tooth to the alveolar bone. Here cementum on the surface of the root (left) is fused with the alveolar bone (right).

**179 Reimplanted teeth.** External resorption of the root can occur after a tooth has been reimplanted in its socket. This unexplained sequela is a cause of failure of the operation.

# (iii) Defects of structure

**180 Amelogenesis imperfecta.** Hypoplasia. Minor defects in hypoplasia result in the formation of pits or grooves of the enamel surface.

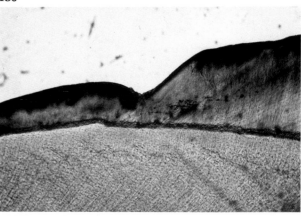
180

**181 Amelogenesis imperfecta.** Hypoplasia. Thin glassy enamel in markedly hypoplastic enamel with an almost total absence of rod structure.

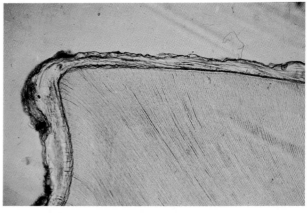
181

**182 Amelogenesis imperfecta.** Hypomaturation. A mild hypomineralisation which morphologically shows normal enamel thickness and rod structure.

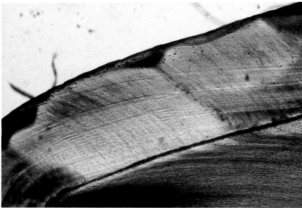
182

**183 Amelogenesis imperfecta.** Hypomaturation. Polarised light and first order red plate. Hypomineralised areas with large areas of positive birefringence are highlighted. Same field as **182**.

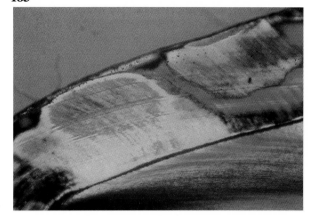

**184 Amelogenesis imperfecta.** Hypomineralisation. In hypomineralised varieties of amelogenesis imperfecta, the enamel matrix is often acid-resistant and remain as caps following demineralisation of the teeth.

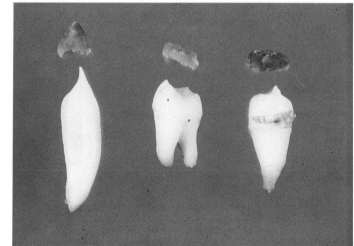

**185 Amelogenesis imperfecta.** Hypomineralisation. Paraffin sections of this retained enamel matrix show the presence of repetitious deposition of cuticular material on the surface of the enamel.

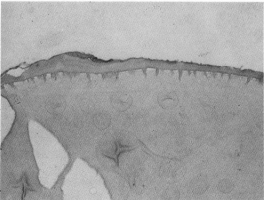

**193**

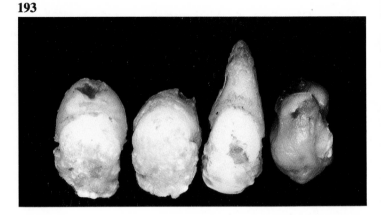

**193 Odontodysplasia.** Macroscopic appearance of teeth affected by this condition. The teeth look malformed and markedly hypoplastic. The roots are often poorly formed.

**194 Odontodysplasia.** A radiograph shows the ghostly appearance of the teeth. This is not always attained and often the teeth merely look hypoplastic.

**195 Odontodysplasia.** The coronal dentine exhibits an amorphous basophilic area that is devoid of collagen and contains cellular inclusions.

**196 Odontodysplasia.** The pulp chamber remains large and root development is often retarded, accounting for the ghostly appearance on radiographs. Pulp stones are frequent.

**194**

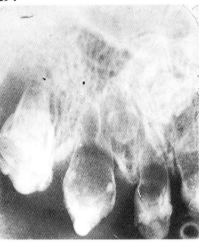

**195**

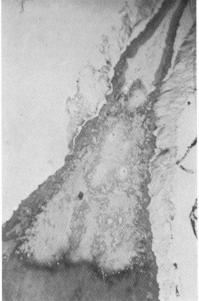

**196**

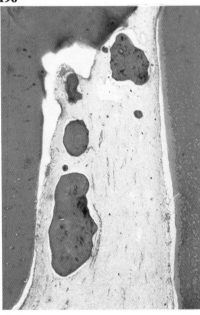

**197**

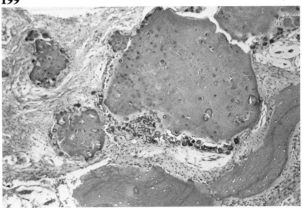

**197 Odontodysplasia.** Parts of the dentine may show marked interglobular dentine formation.

**198**

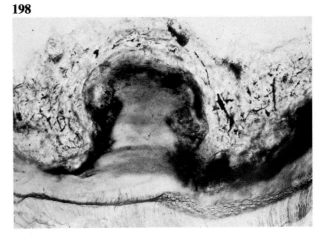

**198 Odontodysplasia.** The enamel is hypoplastic with alternate areas of prismatic enamel and glassy mineralisation.

**199**

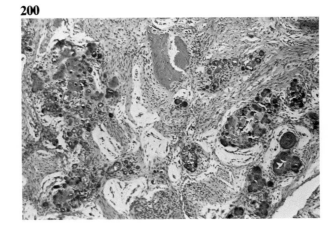

**199 Odontodysplasia.** Within the follicle surrounding the unerupted tooth are cementum-like masses, which have been referred to as Type B calcification, and foci of particulate calcification. Strands and islands of odontogenic epithelium are also present.

**200 Odontodysplasia.** Foci of particulate calcification within the follicles of odontodysplastic teeth have been referred to as Type A calcification.

**200**

**201**

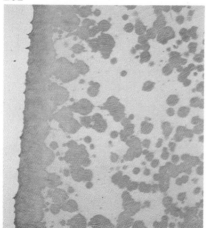

**202**

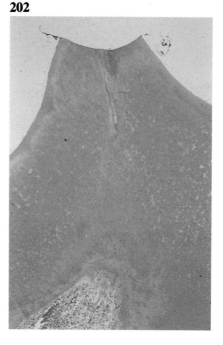

**201 Rickets.** Large areas of interglobular dentine are seen in the dentine.

**202 Vitamin D resistant rickets.** In addition to the areas of interglobular dentine, some teeth show the presence of a slender pulp horn which extends to the amelodentinal junction. Direct bacterial ingress following eruption and attrition of the occlusal surface results in pulp death and presentation as alveolar abscess in apparently non-carious teeth.

**203**

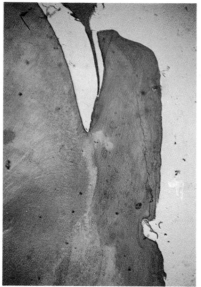

**204**

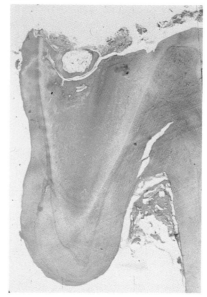

**203 Hypercementosis.** An increase in thickness of the cementum layer may be idiopathic in origin, such as the case in buried teeth.

**204 Hypercementosis of roots of teeth as a manifestation of Paget's disease.** There may be hypercementosis of the roots of the entire dentition in Paget's disease. The excessive remodelling may even result in the formation of a mosaic pattern in the cementum.

**205**

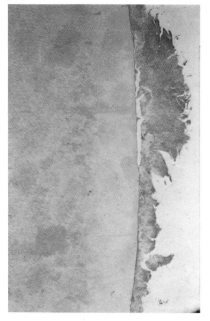

**206**

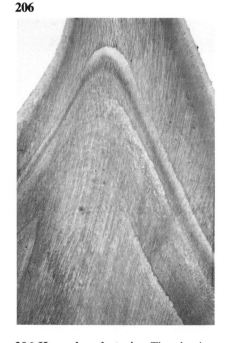

**205 Hypophosphatasia.** Failure of cementum formation in this condition results in loosening of the teeth, particularly involving the deciduous dentition. The exposed dentine surface is covered heavily with bacterial plaque.

**206 Hypophosphatasia.** The dentine may show prominent incremental lines, indicating the disturbance in dentinogenesis.

**207 Cleido-cranial dysplasia.** Cellular cementum is normally found covering the apical halves of the root surfaces. In many cases of cleido-cranial dysplasia, it is markedly deficient and acellular cementum covers the entire root. *(Picrothionin)*

**207**

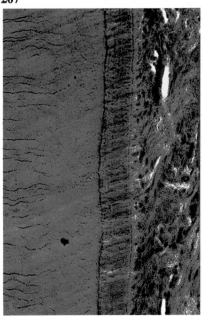

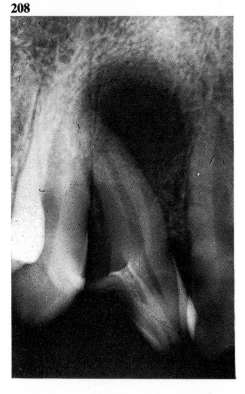

**208**

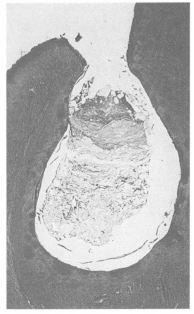

**209**

**210**

**208 Dens invaginatus.** This condition usually affects the maxillary lateral incisor and the invagination commences at the lingual pit. It is often diagnosed radiographically as an enamel-lined pit which may be dilated at the base.

**209 Dens invaginatus.** Radiograph of a specimen of dens invaginatus which has resulted in a dilated root end. Such anomalies have been referred to as dilated odontomes.

**210 Dens invaginatus.** Histologically, the invagination is lined with enamel. However, this enamel lining is often deficient at the base and patent dentinal tubules are exposed to the oral environment, allowing direct bacterial ingress to the pulp to take place.

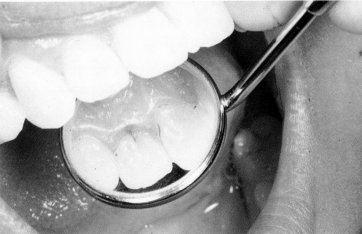

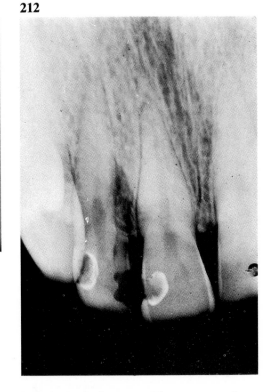

**211 Palato-gingival groove.** This is a developmental defect which may affect any of the maxillary incisor teeth, although the maxillary lateral incisor is the most commonly affected. The defect takes the form of a groove between the cingulum and one of the lateral marginal ridges, and courses along the surface of the root. This is a predisposing cause of localised periodontal disease.

**212 Palato-gingival groove.** The presence of the groove may be visualised as a radiolucent line coursing down the root surface.

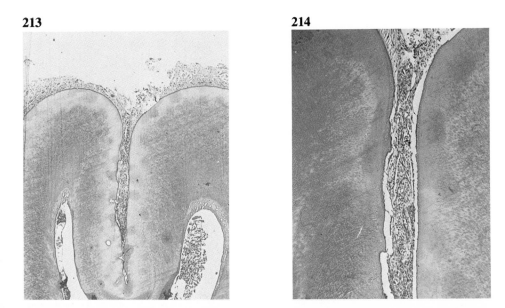

**213 Palato-gingival groove.** When the tooth is involved, granulation tissue diffusely infiltrated with inflammatory cells fills the groove and the pulp may be secondarily involved.

**214 Palato-gingival groove.** Higher power view of the groove which is filled with granulation tissue.

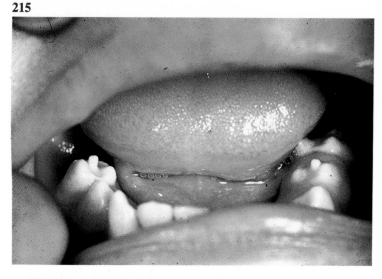

**215 Dens evaginatus.** This is the antithesis of dens invaginatus. The teeth affected are usually the premolars. There is a tubercle on the occlusal surface and, when the tooth is erupted, the tubercle undergoes attrition, or fracture. There is often a pulp horn within the tubercle; direct exposure of the pulp or direct invasion of the pulp via the patent dentinal tubules by micro-organisms takes place, resulting in pulp death.

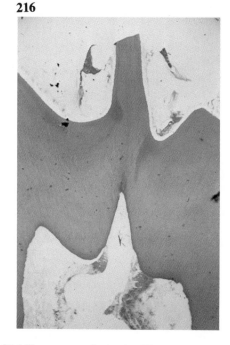

**216 Dens evaginatus.** Histologically, there is often extension of the pulp horn for a variable distance into the tubercle. Following exposure of patent dentinal tubules, if not actual exposure of the pulp extension, direct bacterial ingress leads to pulp death.

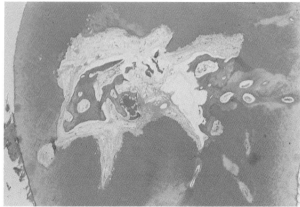

**217 Idiopathic internal resorption.** In this form of idiopathic resorption, the tooth presents as a 'pink-spot'. Concomitant repair accompanies the process of resorption.

**218 Tetracycline staining.** The staining of dental tissues by the antibiotic is best visualised by examination of ground sections with ultraviolet light. Yellow fluorescent lines are seen, usually in the dentine, but all the calcified dental tissues may show its presence.

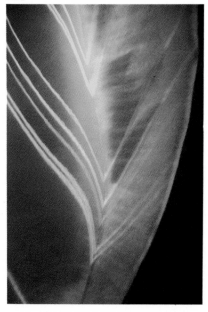

# (iv) Gingivitis and chronic inflammatory periodontal disease

**219**

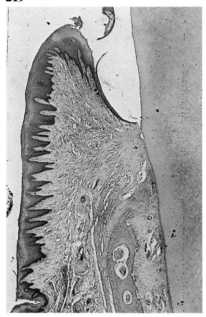

**219 Normal tissues of the periodontium.** The tissues of the periodontium comprise the gingiva, periodontal ligament, alveolar bone and cementum. In the young adult the free gingiva hugs the neck of the tooth and crevice depth is minimal.

**220**

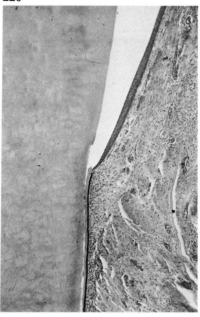

**220 Junctional epithelium.** This is the remains of the dental organ and terminates at the amelo-cemental junction.

**221**

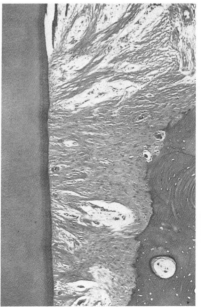

**221 Periodontal ligament, cementum and alveolar bone.** Free gingival fibres which run from the cementum to the gingiva, alveolar crest fibres which run to the crest of the alveolus and horizontal fibres are three principal groups of fibres seen here.

**222 Bundle bone of the alveolus, periodontal ligament and cementum.** Bundle bone of the alveolus, so-called because the principal fibres of the periodontal ligament are attached to it by bundles of Sharpey's fibres, is a type of bone peculiar to the tooth socket. It often shows many resting lines as a reflection of the remodelling activity that occurs as a result of the physiological movement of the tooth. The oblique fibres which run from the alveolar bone to the cementum show that this is a deeper part of the socket.

**222**

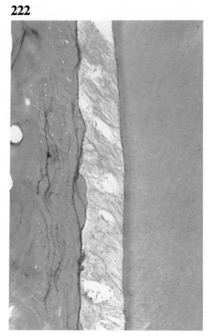

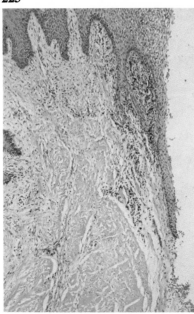

**223**

**223 Early gingivitis.** Accumulation of lymphocytes is seen close to the junctional epithelium.

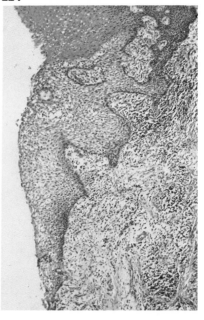

**224**

**224 Early gingivitis.** The junctional epithelium exhibits marked spongiosis, and polymorphonuclear leucocyte infiltration.

**225 The masticatory gingiva.** This is the part of the gingiva which is subject to masticatory activity. It includes both the free and attached gingiva, and is normally covered with a keratinized or parakeratinized stratified squamous epithelium. The lamina propria is free from inflammatory cell infiltration in early gingivitis.

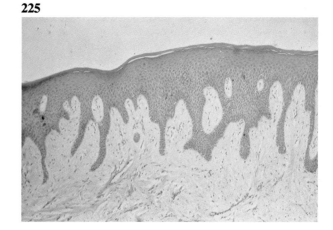

**226 Late gingivitis.** As the inflammatory process spreads, the lamina propria of the gingiva is diffusely infiltrated with lymphocytes and plasma cells. The covering stratified squamous epithelium loses its keratin layer and becomes non-keratinized.

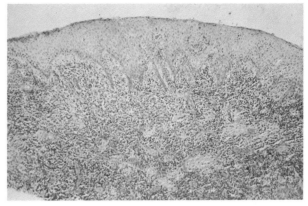

**227 Gingival abscess.** An acute inflammatory reaction which becomes localised in the gingiva may give rise to abscess formation with a heavy aggregation of polymorphonuclear leucocytes in the gingiva.

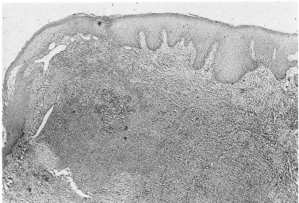

**228 Resorption of alveolar bone.** Resorption of alveolar bone by osteoclastic activity may be seen as a gradual reduction of height of the alveolar crest, giving rise to 'horizontal resorption' or an increase in thickness of the periodontal ligament space, resulting in so-called 'vertical resorption'.

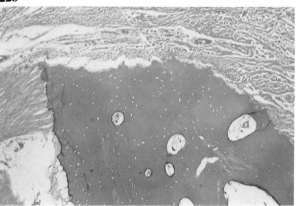

**229 Horizontal resorption of the alveolar crest.** Marked resorption results in the formation of a crater-shaped alveolar crest which can be seen in clinical radiographs.

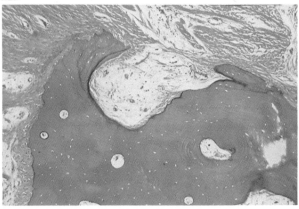

**230 'Vertical resorption' of the alveolar crest.** Osteoclastic resorption of the bundle bone lining the socket results in a thickened periodontal ligament, and is sometimes referred to as 'vertical resorption'.

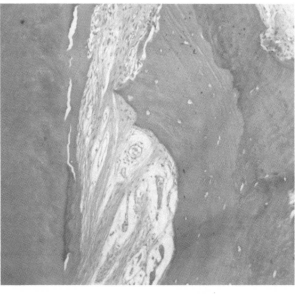

**231**

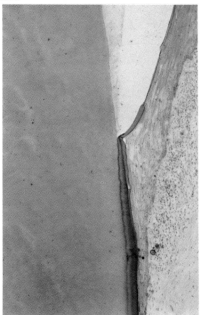

**232**

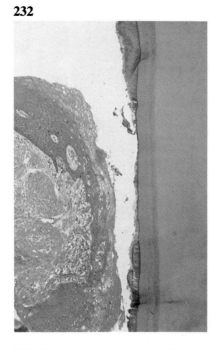

**231 Migration of the junctional epithelium.** As a response to the inflammatory process, the junctional epithelium moves down the surface of the root.

**232 Formation of a periodontal pocket.** In addition to migration down the surface of the root, the junctional epithelium may also develop rete processes. Calculus and bacterial plaque are seen attached to the root surface and the corium is diffusely infiltrated with lymphocytes and plasma cells.

**233 Base of the periodontal pocket.** The junctional epithelium which has migrated down the surface of the root forms the most apical part of the pocket. Granulation tissue diffusely infiltrated with chronic inflammatory cells lie beneath the crevicular epithelium which lines the pocket. Pockets which terminate below the height of the alveolar crest are called 'infra-bony', while those which remain above the crest are called 'supra-bony' pockets.

**233**

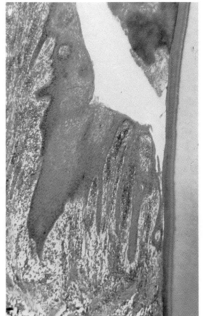

# 5 Cysts of the oral tissues and jaws

**234**

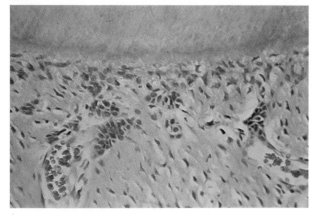

**234 Epithelial rests of Malassez.** These islands of odontogenic epithelium are found scattered in the periodontal ligament. They are part of a network resulting from the disintegration of Hertwig's epithelial sheath.

**235**

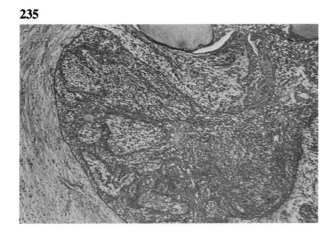

**235 Epithelial proliferation in a periapical granuloma.** When inflammation spreads to the periodontal ligament, usually as an extension of infection from a necrotic pulp, the epithelial rests of Malassez may be stimulated to proliferate.

**236**

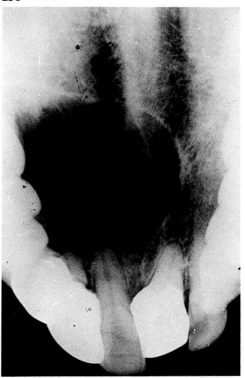

**236 Radicular cyst.** Occlusal radiograph showing a well-circumscribed radiolucent area at the periapical region of a non-vital maxillary lateral incisor.

**237 Radicular cyst.** Cystic change takes place in a periapical granuloma in an undefined manner, resulting in the formation of a cavity lined with non-keratinized stratified squamous epithelium.

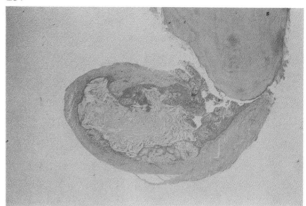

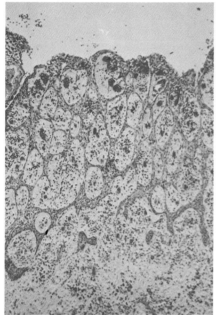

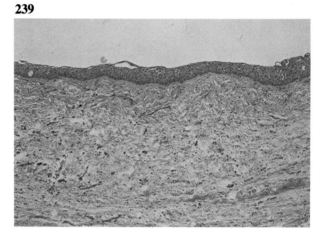

**239 Radicular cyst.** In older cysts, the epithelial lining is usually a thin, non-keratinized stratified squamous epithelium, and the underlying fibrous tissue is less inflamed.

**238 Radicular cyst.** In young cysts, the epithelial lining often proliferates to form arcades or rings around the underlying connective tissue.

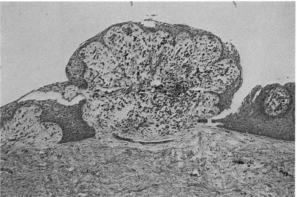

**240 Mural nodule in a cyst lining.** Thickening on the walls of cysts may be composed of granulation tissue diffusely infiltrated with inflammatory cells.

**241**

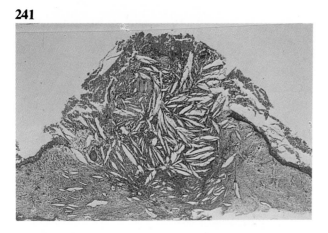

**241 Radicular cyst.** The cyst cavity is filled with an eosinophilic coagulum containing slit-like spaces which contain cholesterol. These cholesterol masses may also form mural nodules; the epithelial lining becomes discontinuous where such nodules have formed.

**242**

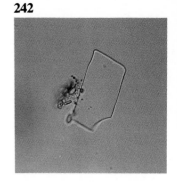

**242 Cholesterol crystal.** Although cholesterol appears as spindle-shaped slits in histological sections, when cyst fluid is examined directly under the microscope it appears as a rhomboid-shaped plate with one corner cut off.

**243 Goblet cell metaplasia.** The mucus-secreting or goblet cells are the result of metaplasia of the non-keratinized stratified squamous epithelium and are stained here with a PAS technique.

**243**

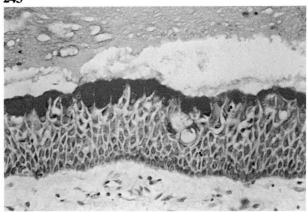

**244 Hyaline bodies.** Another feature that may be seen within the epithelial linings of radicular cysts is the peculiarly shaped structures which are eosiniphilic and, typically, are described as ladies' hair-pin-shaped. There is considerable uncertainty about the nature and origin of these hyaline bodies; various investigators have suggested that they may be keratinous in nature, of hematogenous origin, or that they may be a specialised secretory product of odontogenic epithelium.

**244**

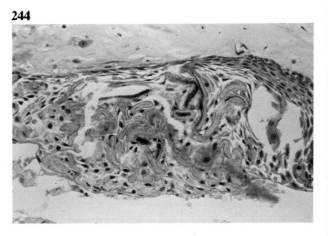

**253**
rega
pres
over
kera
sube
by i

**254**
men
be s
of t
the
is n
with
call

**255**
new
vari
ing
lium
para
seer

**245**

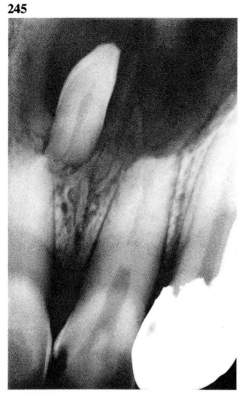

**245 Dentigerous cyst** (follicular cyst). This is a cyst which has enclosed within it the crown of a tooth. In this case the tooth is a supernumerary mesiodens.

**247 Dentigerous cyst.** The typical lining of this cyst is composed of a thin non-keratinized stratified squamous epithelium backed by an uninflamed fibrous tissue.

**248 Goblet and ciliated cell metaplasia in a dentigerous cyst.** As in radicular cysts, goblet and ciliated cells may be seen as a metaplastic change in the epithelial lining of a dentigerous cyst.

**246**

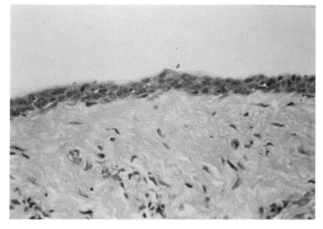

**246 Dentigerous cyst.** The lining of a dentigerous or follicular cyst is attached to the amelocemental junction and the pulp of the associated tooth is vital. This anatomical criterion must be satisfied before a diagnosis of dentigerous cyst is valid.

**247**

**248**

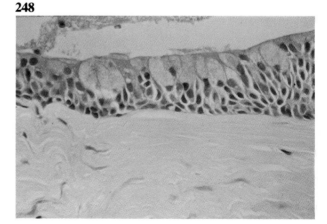

**256**

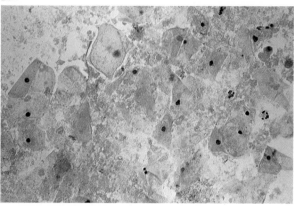

**256 Odontogenic keratocyst** (primordial cyst). Smear preparations from aspirated cyst fluid show large numbers of epithelial squames.

**257**

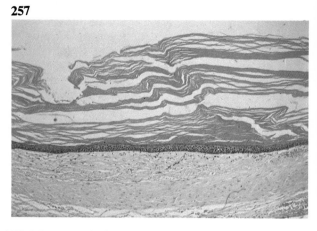

**257 Odontogenic keratocyst** (primordial cyst). The lining of the odontogenic keratocyst is typically a thin lining of keratinized stratified epithelium, backed with uninflamed connective tissue. The cyst cavity is filled with keratin that has been shed by the epithelium.

**258**

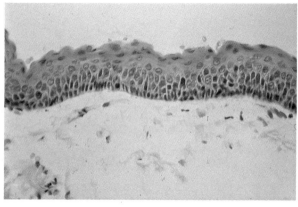

**258 Odontogenic keratocyst** (primordial cyst). The epithelial lining of an odontogenic keratocyst is thin, usually not more than ten cells thick. The surface is more often parakeratinized than orthokeratinized and the epithelial-connective tissue junction is flattened and devoid of rete processes. The underlying connective tissue is typically free from inflammatory cell infiltrate.

**259**

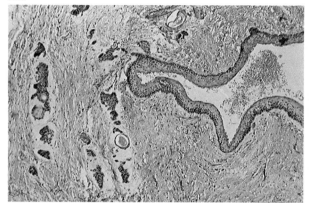

**259 Odontogenic keratocyst** (primordial cyst). In some keratocysts many islands of epithelium are seen in the fibrous wall. They are thought to contribute to the higher rate of recurrence in keratocysts, because of their tendency to form satellite cysts. Cysts associated with the basal cell naevoid syndrome are said to exhibit this feature more frequently than solitary cysts.

**260**

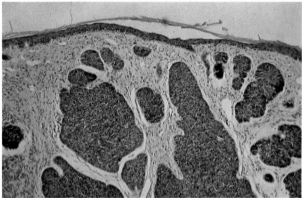

**261**

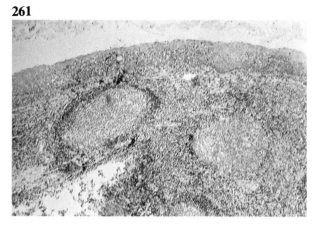

**260 Basal cell naevoid lesion in the skin of a patient with Gorlin's syndrome** (basal cell naevoid syndrome). The basal cell naevoid lesions in the skin are indistinguishable from basal cell carcinoma histologically and may appear at any time from adolescence to the third decade.

**261 Benign lymphoepithelial cyst.** These cysts may be seen also in the soft tissues of the oral cavity. The lining is poorly parakeratinized and there are lymphoid follicles in the fibrous wall.

**262**

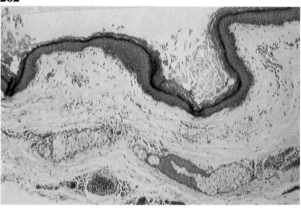

**263**

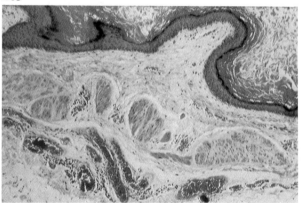

**262 Dermoid cyst.** These cysts are seen usually in the floor of the mouth. The lining of the cyst is a keratinized stratified squamous epithelium and sebaceous glands and hair follicles are present in the fibrous wall.

**263 Dermoid cyst.** Another part of the cyst lining with smooth muscle is present in the wall. Similar cysts without the presence of appendage structures are called epidermoid cysts.

# 6 Epithelial premalignant lesions and neoplasms

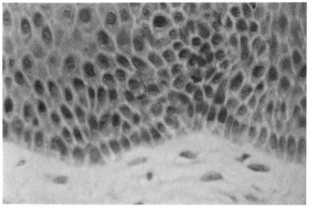

**273 Mucosal epithelium of normal appearance.** The basal cells are polarised at right angles to the epithelial-connective tissue junction and the prickle-cells are arranged in regular stratification from below upwards.

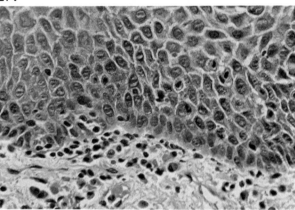

**274 Disturbance of polarity in the basal cell layer.** The basal cells are not perpendicular to the epithelial-connective tissue junction but are positioned at an angle to the junction.

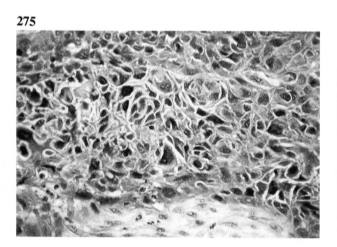

**275 Pleomorphism and hyperchromatism.** The cells show a variation in shape and size and many nuclei are darkly stained.

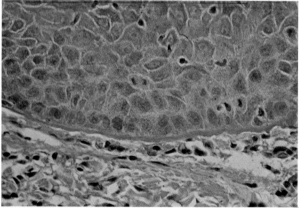

**276 Thickening of the basement membrane.** An increase in thickness in the PAS positive 'basement membrane' may be seen.

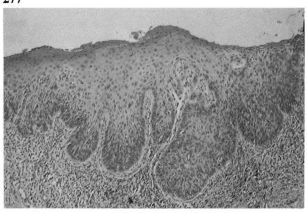

**277 Drop-shaped rete processes.** The rete processes become irregular, often with a bulbous basal portion and a constriction higher up.

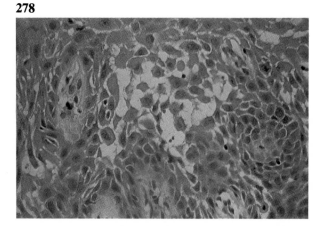

**278 Loss of cohesion.** The prickle-cells lose their attachment to their neighbouring cells with an appearance similar to acantholysis.

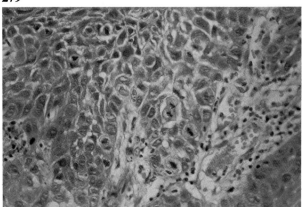

**279 Increased mitoses.** Increased mitotic activity can be seen in premalignant and malignant lesions. Mitosis at a high prickle-cell level is particularly important.

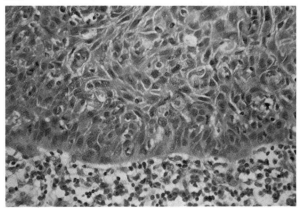

**280 Marked disturbance in polarity.** The disturbance in cellular arrangement is more marked and the regular stratification in the prickle-cell layer is replaced by cells arranged irregularly.

**289**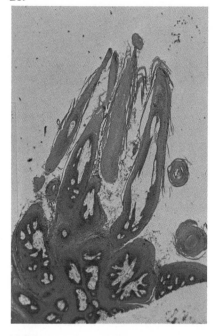

**290**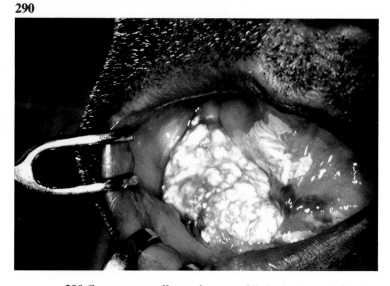

**290 Squamous cell carcinoma.** Clinical photograph of a fungating squamous cell carcinoma that has developed on the alveolar mucosa adjacent to a sublingual keratosis.

**289 Squamous papilloma.** The lesion is composed of multiple finger-like processes, each covered with a keratinized or parakeratinized stratified squamous epithelium with a connective tissue core.

**291**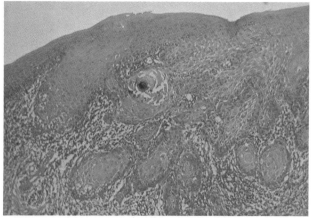

**291 Squamous cell carcinoma.** The neoplastic epithelium is of surface origin and strands and islands of the tumour are invading the connective tissue. A diffuse chronic inflammatory cell infiltrate accompanies the epithelial prolongations. A small edge of normal mucosa can be seen.

**292 Squamous cell carcinoma.** Islands of neoplastic epithelium have invaded the connective tissue. Several keratin whorls (cell nests) are seen.

**292**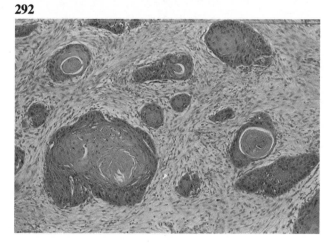

**293 Squamous cell carcinoma.** Epithelial strands displaying pleomorphism and hyperchromatism are within the connective tissue. There are no cell nests but the degree of differentation is still fairly high.

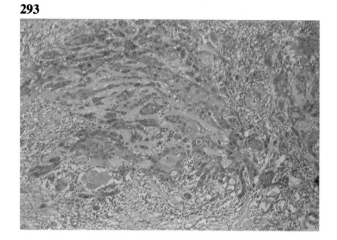

**293**

**294 Squamous cell carcinoma.** In this carcinoma, the tumour is poorly differentiated. The cytological features of malignancy are marked; there is little or no evidence of keratin formation.

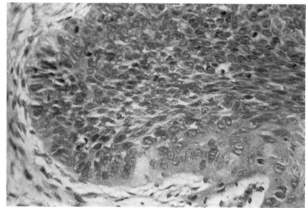

**294**

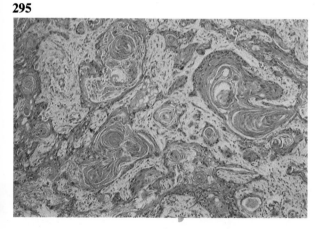

**295**

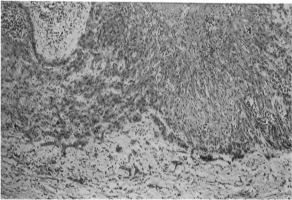

**296**

**295 and 296 Squamous cell carcinoma.** The difficulty in grading the degree of differentiation of a tumour can be appreciated in these two photomicrographs which are from two fields of the same tumour.

Figure **295** shows marked cell nest formation, while in **296**, the tumour is less well differentiated.

**297**

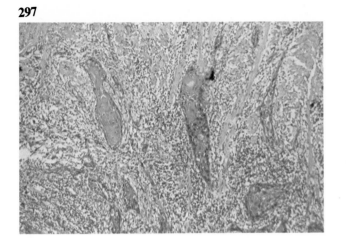

**297 Invasion by squamous cell carcinoma.** The tumour has invaded the underlying muscle.

**298**

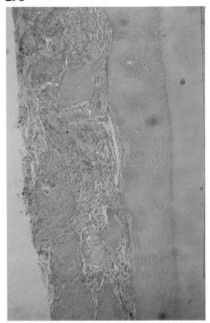

**298 Squamous cell carcinoma invading the periodontal ligament.** Islands of neoplastic epithelium have infiltrated the periodontal ligament alongside the tooth.

**299 Invasion by squamous cell carcinoma.** The tumour has invaded an area of mucous glands.

**299**

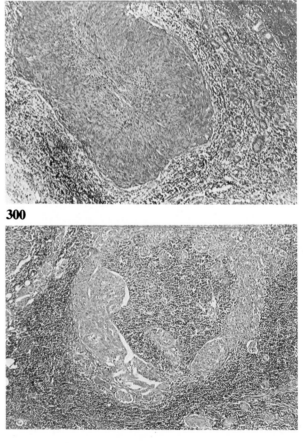

**300 Lymph node metastasis.** The tumour has metastasized to the regional lymph nodes.

**300**

**301**

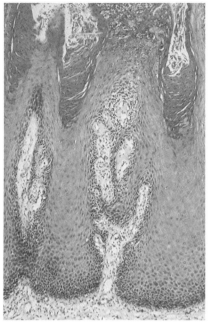

**301 Verrucous carcinoma.** The epithelial prolongations are superficial and tend to be exophytic. The epithelium is deceptively benign in appearance and there is either a hyperkeratosis or hyperparakeratosis.

**303 Epithelial dysplasia.** The cytological features described separately are seen throughout a greater part of the epithelium. The border-line between severe epithelial dysplasia and carcinoma-in-situ is indistinct.

**302**

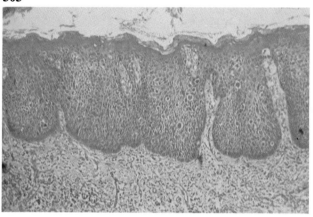

**302 Verrucous hyperplasia.** The surface becomes irregular and papillomatous and a mild to moderate degree of atypia may be apparent in the deeper epithelial cells.

**303**

**304 Carcinoma-in-situ.** The epithelium displays throughout its thickness the features described previously. However, 'top to bottom' change is seen only rarely in oral mucosal lesions.

**304**

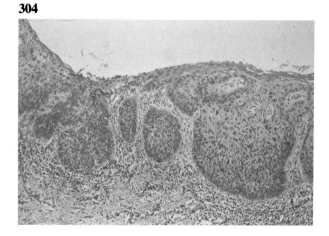

**305**

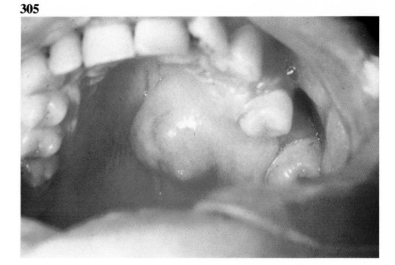

**305 Salivary gland tumour.** The junction of the hard and soft palate is the most common site for intra-oral salivary gland tumours.

**306 Adenolymphoma.** The neoplastic epithelium is twin-layered with many lymphoid follicles in the subepithelial area.

**306**

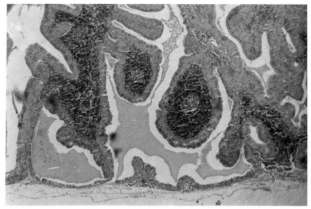

**307 Monomorphic adenoma.** Canalicular type. The neoplastic epithelium is either twin-layered or consists of a single layer of cuboidal cells forming a regular network.

**307**

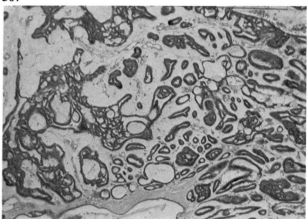

**308 Pleomorphic adenoma.** The neoplasm is composed of sheets of glandular epithelial cells forming duct-like structures containing an eosinophilic secretion.

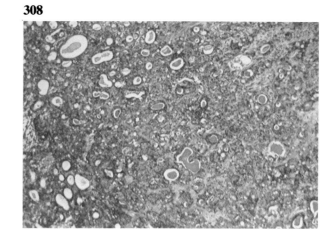

**309 Pleomorphic adenoma.** Higher power view of the tumour epithelial cells and duct-like structures.

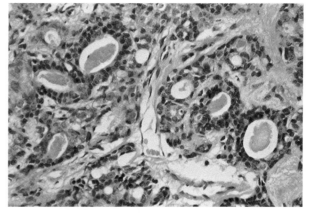

**310 Pleomorphic adenoma.** Separating the more solid tumour epithelial cells is a stroma of fibrous and myxochondroid connective tissue.

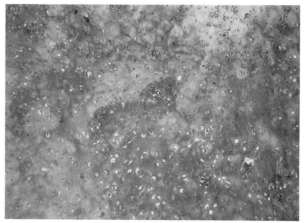

**311 Pleomorphic adenoma.** A more recently recognised feature of the tumour is cells resembling plasma cells – so-called plasmacytoid cells.

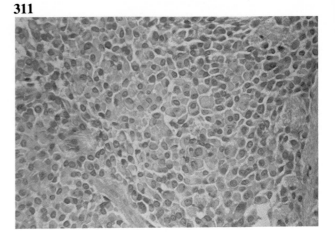

**312 Pleomorphic adenoma.** Squamous metaplasia. Structures resembling cell nests may be seen within some of the duct-like structures.

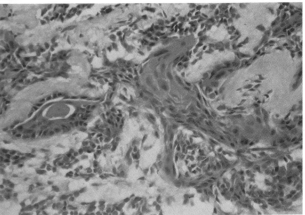

**313 Pleomorphic adenoma.** The presence of a capsule at the periphery is a variable finding in pleomorphic adenomas. In this case, a fibrous capsule has formed.

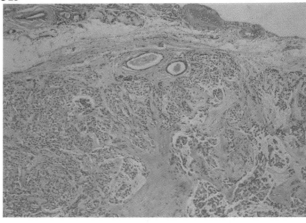

**314 Mucoepidermoid tumour.** The neoplasm is composed of islands of tumour cells which have the characteristics of mucus-secreting cells and epidermoid cells.

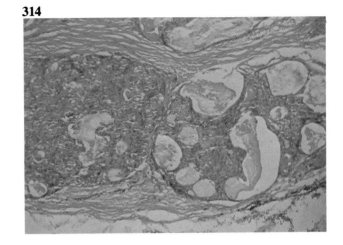

**315 Mucoepidermoid tumour.** Cystic spaces are often seen in the tumour.

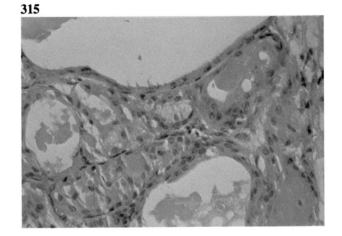

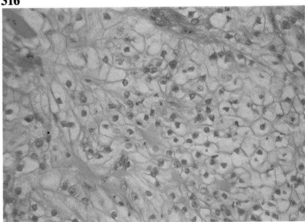

**316 Mucoepidermoid tumour.** Clear cells may be a prominent feature in mucoepidermoid tumour. They do not stain with mucicarmine or fat stains, but may contain glycogen.

**317**

Islands of epithelial cells with 'cystic' spaces.

**317 Adenoid cystic carcinoma.** Islands of epithelial cells with 'cystic' spaces, giving a 'Swiss-cheese' pattern.

**318**

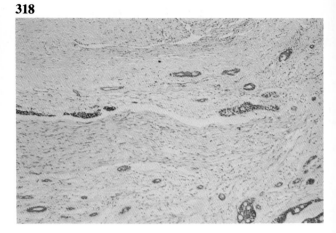

**318 Adenoid cystic carcinoma.** Perineural spread. One of the preferred modes of spread of this tumour is along the course of a peripheral nerve.

**319 Adenocarcinoma.** Islands of epithelial cells with duct-like structures invading normal tissues. Cytological features of malignancy are often seen, although the degree of anaplasia varies.

**319**

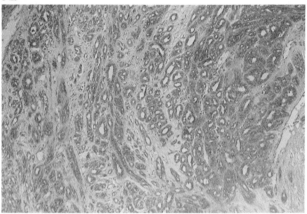

**320 Adenocarcinoma.** The tumour is in close juxtaposition to the overlying epithelium. There is no evidence of a capsule.

**320**

**321 Metastatic carcinoma.** This tumour in the mandible of a 53-year-old woman is a malignant epithelial tumour. A breast carcinoma was removed two years previously. There is marked periosteal new bone deposition.

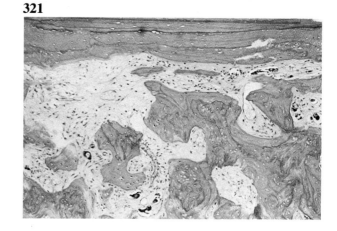

**322 Metastatic carcinoma.** Higher power view of the neoplastic epithelial islands, displaying pleomorphism and hyperchromatism.

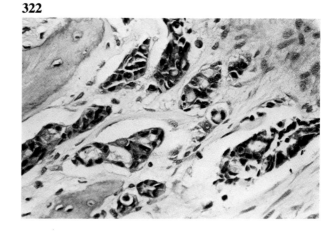

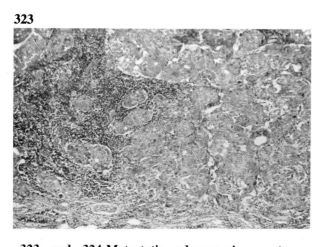

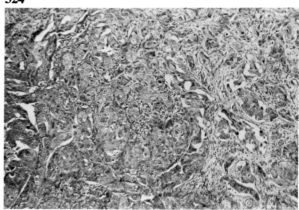

**323 and 324 Metastatic adenocarcinoma (unknown primary).** This tumour presented as a submandibular swelling in a 50-year-old man. The histology is that of an adenocarcinoma in a lymph node. Despite extensive investigations, the search for a primary proved unsuccessful.

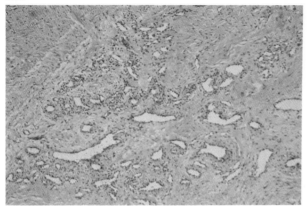

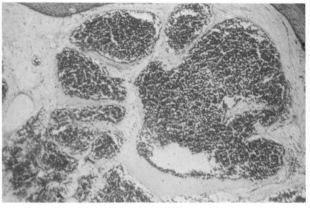

**331 Haemangioma, capillary.** Haemangiomas are developmental anomalies and not neoplasms. There are two principal histological types, capillary and cavernous. Both are lined by a single layer of endothelial cells. This is a capillary haemangioma of the gingiva.

**332 Haemangioma, cavernous.** Here the lumen is a large cavernous space. Surrounding the blood cells is a thin lining of endothelial cells.

**333 Haemangioma** – phlebolith formation. One of the sequelae of oral haemangiomas is thrombosis and phlebolith formation. A laminated calcified mass, the result of an organised thrombus, is seen here.

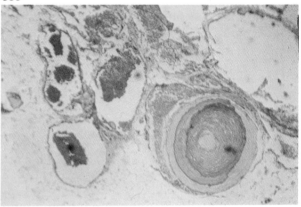

**334 Lymphangioma.** Lymphangiomas are also developmental anomalies. They are composed of spaces filled with pink-staining lymph, and lined with a thin, delicate endothelial lining. They may present as diffuse enlargements of the lip or tongue, or as cystic swellings in the neck, a cystic hygroma. They may also present as small vesicle-like swellings in the oral mucosa, by virtue of their superficial position. The large lymphatic spaces lie just beneath the covering epithelium and may be confused with bullous lesions.

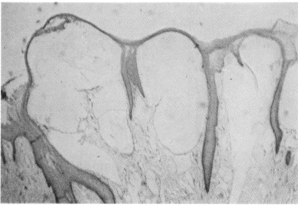

**335**

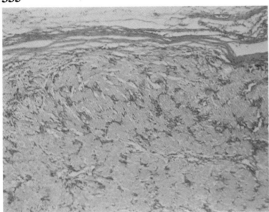

**336**

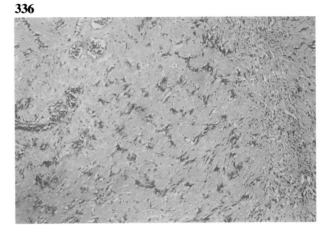

**335 Neurilemmoma.** (Schwannoma). This is a benign neoplasm of Schwann cell origin and is associated with a peripheral nerve. It is encapsulated with a defined band of condensed fibrous tissue at the periphery.

**336 Neurilemmoma.** The histology of the lesion is characteristic. Areas exhibiting palisading of nuclei forming 'Verocay bodies' are referred to as Antoni type A tissue.

**337 Neurilemmoma.** Other areas of the tumour are composed of loose connective tissue without distinctive features. These are referred to as Antoni type B tissue.

**337**

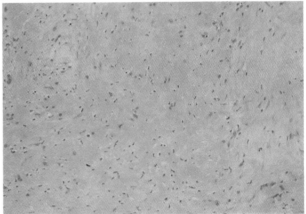

**338 Neurofibroma.** The neurofibroma is not a neoplasm but a developmental anomaly. It may exist as part of von Recklinghausen's multiple neurofibromatosis, or as a solitary lesion. It exhibits a tendency to malignant change. Histologically, it is unencapsulated and consists of spindle-shaped cells and intercellular collagen. Slender nerves are present but are not found easily.

**338**

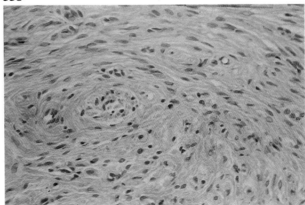

**347 Ossifying fibroma.** This is a benign neoplasm in the jaws. The lesional tissue is a
spindle-cell tumour which exhibits foci of calcification which may range from densely haema-
toxyphilic acellular cementum-like material to
trabeculae of woven bone.

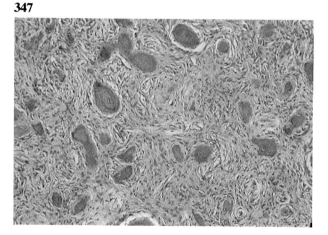

347

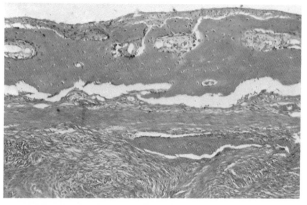

348

**348 Ossifying fibroma.** At the periphery there
may or may not be a capsule of condensed fibrous
tissue. Such a capsule is present here.

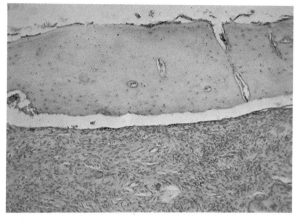

349

**349 Ossifying fibroma.** There is no capsule here
but the lesion is well circumscribed.

**350 Ossifying fibroma.** Trabeculae of woven
bone are seen within the fibrous tissue.

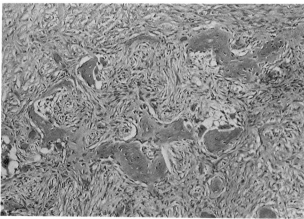

350

**351**

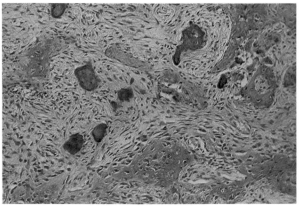

**351 Juvenile ossifying fibroma.** This is a variant of ossifying fibroma affecting younger individuals. As in the adult lesion, both cementum-like material and woven bone may be seen. It is more aggressive in behaviour, and may or may not possess a capsule at the periphery.

**352**

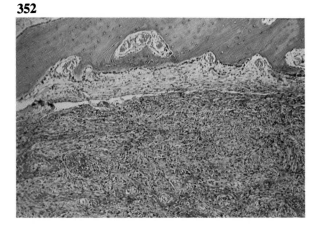

**352 Juvenile ossifying fibroma.** This lesion is well circumscribed at the periphery, but there is no condensed band of fibrous tissue forming a capsule.

**353 Juvenile ossifying fibroma.** Marked osteoclastic activity is a prominent finding, often giving an appearance of complete resorption of a bony trabecula.

**353**

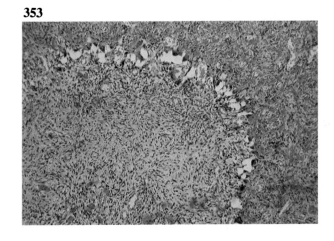

**354 Juvenile ossifying fibroma.** The neurovascular bundle has been displaced to the buccal side of the mandible by the tumour.

**354**

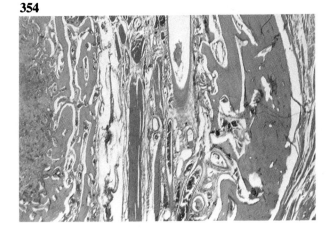

**355**

**356**

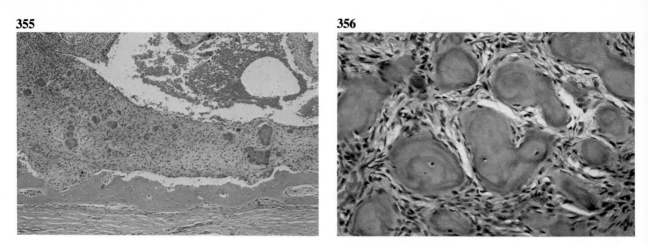

**355 and 356 Aneurysmal bone cyst in association with an ossifying fibroma.** In some cases, the aneurysmal bone cysts may occur in association with other bony lesions. In the jaw bones this is usually an ossifying or cementifying fibroma. Such lesions tend to behave more aggressively, either growing to a huge size causing marked facial deformity, or exhibiting a greater tendency to recurrence.

**357**

**358**

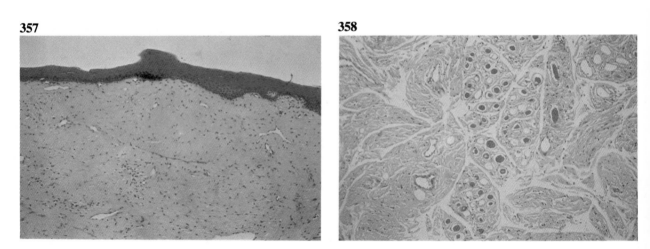

**357 and 358 Amyloid tumour.** Amyloid deposits may be found in oral tissues, usually in the tongue. Sometimes they may appear as discrete tumours, while at other times they present as diffuse enlargements of the tongue. They may be primary or secondary in origin, in the latter case usually following myelomatosis. This was an amyloidosis secondary to myeloma.

**359 Chondroma.** This is a rare tumour in the jaws, but may be seen in the premaxillary region or in the condyle of the mandible. The lesion is composed of a mass of cartilage of normal appearance.

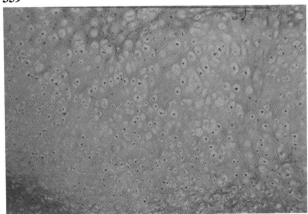

**360 Osteomas.** These are bony masses which form either subperiosteally or as endosteal lesions; most are developmental abnormalities and it is doubtful if any are neoplastic. They may occur as part of Gardner's syndrome, together with polyposis of the colon and epidermoid cysts and fibromas of the skin. Histologically they are of two varieties. Shown here is the compact or ivory osteoma which is composed of a mass of compact bone with haversian systems.

**360**

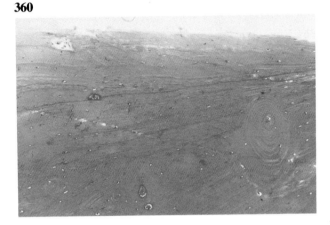

**361 Osteoma.** The other histological variety of osteoma is the cancellous osteoma which is made up of trabeculae of cancellous bone with haemopoietic or fatty marrow between the trabeculae. Oral tori and exostoses are indistinguishable histologically from osteomas.

**361**

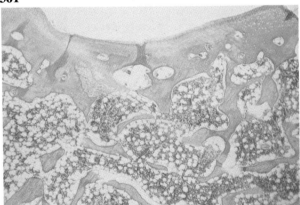

**370**

**371**

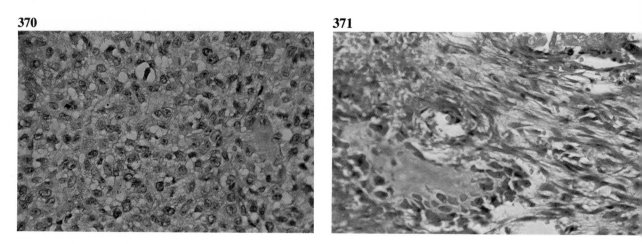

**370 and 371 Osteosarcoma.** In osteosarcoma the malignant mesenchyme produces osteoid and mineralised bone which may vary in appearance.

**372**

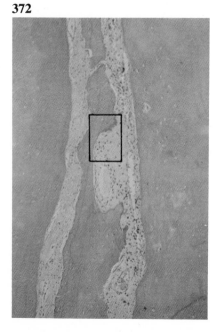

**373**

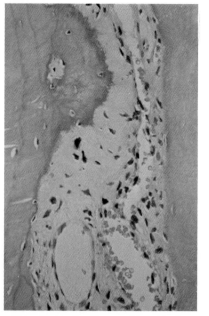

**372 Osteosarcoma.** In the tooth-bearing part of the jaws, thickening of the periodontal membrane shadow around teeth without evidence of local-ised disease is often an important radiographic sign. The histological evidence of periodontal involvement by the tumour in the bifurcation of a mandibular molar is shown here.

**373 Osteosarcoma.** Higher power view (of boxed area in **372**) showing malignant mesenchyme, producing osteoid and abnormal tumour bone in the periodontal ligament.

**374 Osteosarcoma** – parosteal. This is a special variant of osteosarcoma which is of periosteal origin and has a better prognosis than the central variety. The cytological evidence of malignancy is minimal and the tumour bone formed is usually well differentiated.

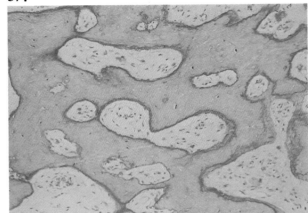

**375 Malignant lymphoma** (non-Hodgkin's). Because of the complexity and lack of uniformity in classification of this group of malignant tumours, only selective examples of oral interest are illustrated. This is a follicular type of centro-blastic-centrocytic malignant lymphoma (Kiel classification).

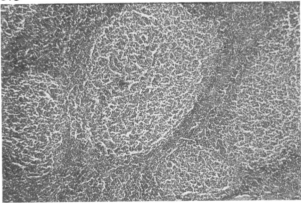

**376 Burkitt's lymphoma.** This form of malignant lymphoma chiefly occurs in children in a geographically defined belt in Africa. The tumour affects multiple quadrants in the jaws as well as paired organs, and is composed of primitive lymphoid cells of B cell origin. Non-neoplastic histiocytes are scattered among the tumour cells, giving the 'starry sky' appearance. This appearance, however, is not pathognomonic of Burkitt's lymphoma.

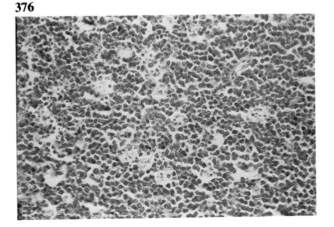

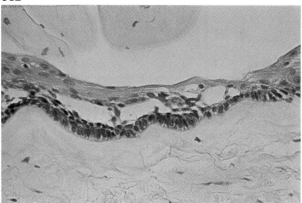

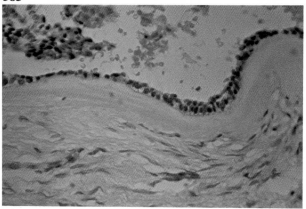

**382 Ameloblastoma** – cystic area. The cells lining the cystic area of an ameloblastoma may be columnar or cuboidal dark-staining cells betraying their neoplastic nature.

**383 Ameloblastoma** – cystic area. In the cystic area the tumour may be lined by an epithelium that resembles a non-neoplastic cyst. A hyalinised band of collagen is sometimes seen subepithelially. It may be mistaken for induction.

**384 Ameloblastoma** – squamous metaplasia. The stellate reticulum-like cells in the central part of the islands may assume an epidermoid or squamous appearance with formation of prickle-cells and keratin.

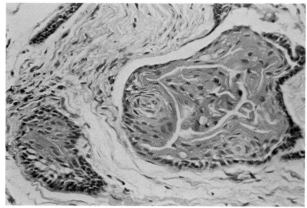

**385 Ameloblastoma** – plexiform type. This is the other common histological appearance of an ameloblastoma. Strands of odontogenic epithelium ramify in a fibrous connective tissue matrix giving an appearance of connective tissue 'follicles' in an epithelial 'stroma'.

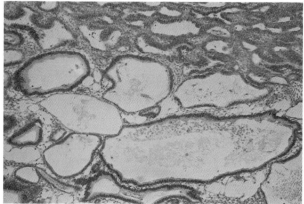

**386 Peripheral ameloblastoma.** Very rarely an extra-osseous ameloblastoma may present as an epulis, indistinguishable clinically from the inflammatory epulides. The histology is identical to the intra-osseous lesion, although biologically it appears to have a more innocuous behaviour, simple excision being curative.

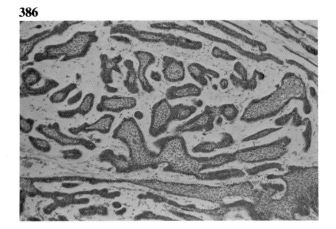

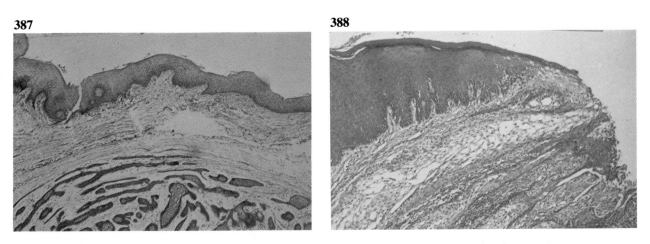

**387 and 388 Peripheral ameloblastoma.** The lesional tissue sometimes is not connected to the covering mucosa, as in this instance. At other times fusion with the covering epithelium may suggest a surface origin.

**389 Ameloblastoma** – granular cell type. The stellate reticulum-like cells may undergo a granular cell change.

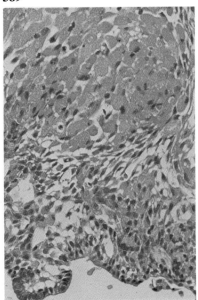

**390 Calcifying epithelial odontogenic tumour**
(Pindborg tumour). The tumour is composed of
sheets of polyhedral squamous cells in a fibrous
stroma. Eosinophilic globules exhibiting the
staining characteristics of amyloid are prominent
among the tumour foci.

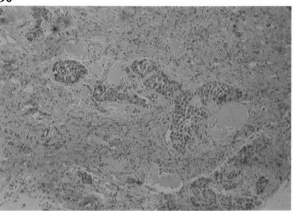

**391 Calcifying epithelial odontogenic tumour**
(Pindborg tumour). Cellular pleomorphism is
marked but the clinical behaviour of the lesion is,
at worst, locally invasive.

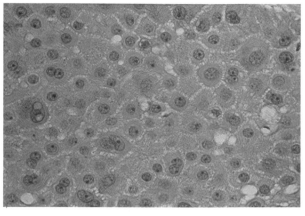

**392 Calcifying epithelial odontogenic tumour**
(Pindborg tumour). The eosinophilic globules
may be shown to exhibit thioflavine-T
fluorescence.

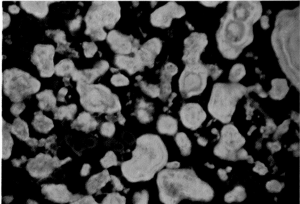

**393 Adenomatoid odontogenic tumour** (adeno-ameloblastoma). The lesion often presents as a dentigerous cyst with a well-circumscribed radiolucent area around the crown of a buried tooth. Small flecks of radiopaque material are seen within the radiolucent area, often separated by a radiolucent zone from a radiopaque margin.

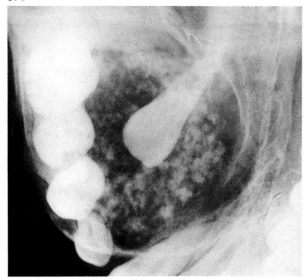

**394 Adenomatoid odontogenic tumour.** The macroscopic appearance of the lesion corresponds to the radiographic appearance with a well-formed fibrous capsule enveloping the lesional tissue and the crown of the buried tooth.

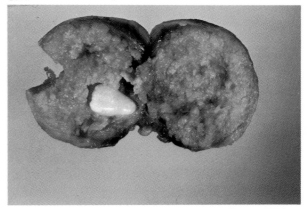

**395 Adenomatoid odontogenic tumour.** The typical histology of the lesion contains duct-like structures lined with tall columnar cells and lobules of spindle- or polyhedral cells in a scanty fibrous stroma which is often haemorrhagic.

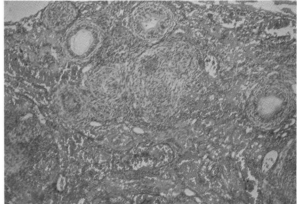

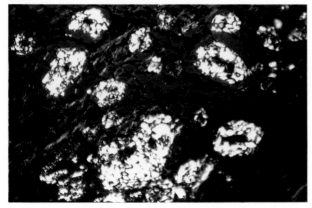

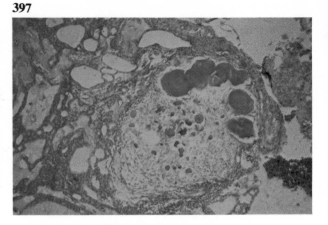

**396 Adenomatoid odontogenic tumour.** Eosinophilic globules are seen within the epithelial masses. They exhibit the staining characteristics of amyloid. *(Alkaline Congo red, polarised light)*

**397 Adenomatoid odontogenic tumour.** Less commonly, there are areas of dentine or cementum-like material, indicating that an inductive process is present.(*van Gieson*)

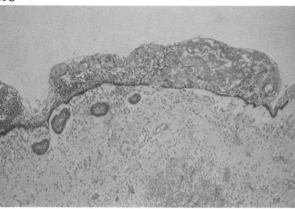

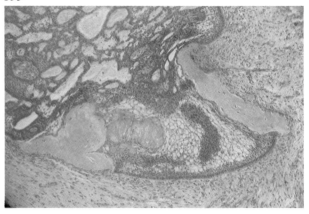

**398 Calcifying odontogenic cyst.** The typical histology is that of an epithelial cyst with tall columnar cells at the periphery and masses of ghost cells within. 'Dysplastic dentine' may also have been induced.

**399 Calcifying odontogenic cyst** – peripheral lesion. Very rarely, epulides showing the histology of calcifying odontogenic cysts are also seen. They are solid lesions and behave in a benign fashion.

**400**

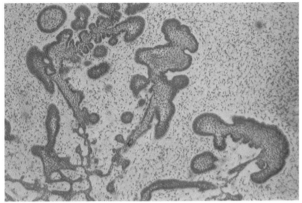

**400 Ameloblastic fibroma.** The lesion is a neoplasm behaving like an ameloblastoma, contrary to the belief that it is more benign. It is composed of strands of odontogenic epithelium in a stroma that strongly resembles dental papilla.

**401**

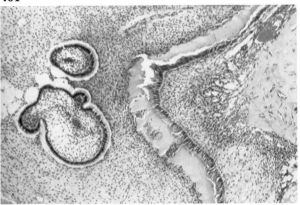

**401 Ameloblastic fibro-odontoma.** This is a lesion in which both soft and hard dental tissues are formed simultaneously. The soft component is similar to an ameloblastic fibroma, with strands and islands of odontogenic epithelium and a dental papilla-like stroma. In addition, dentine and enamel are formed.

**402**

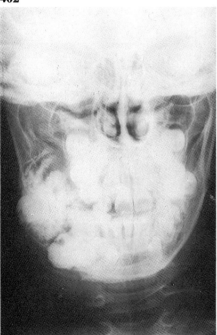

**402 Complex odontome.** Posterior–anterior radiograph showing an irregular radiopaque mass in the right mandible.

**403**

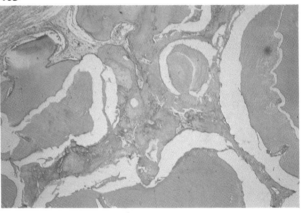

**403 Complex odontome.** An irregular mass of all the formed dental tissues in haphazard arrangement is seen. Enamel, dentine, pulp and cementum are all identifiable.

**404 Compound odontome.** Definite tooth-like structures are formed and the arrangement of the dental tissues is much more regular than the complex odontome. Examples intermediate in appearance are not uncommon and are then called complex or compound, according to the predominance of the component.

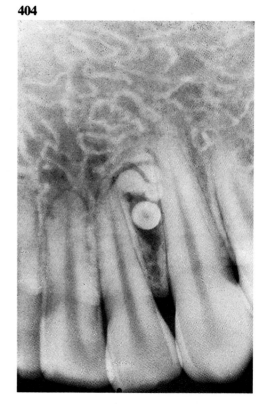

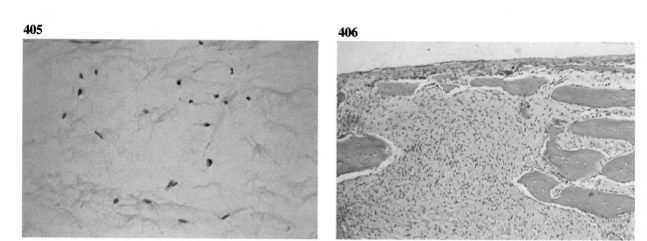

**405 and 406 Odontogenic myxoma.** The tumour is composed of undifferentiated mesenchymel cells resembling those in Wharton's jelly. They may be stellate or angular in addition to being spindle-shaped. Relatively little collagen is elaborated and much glycosaminoglycans is present in the stroma. The lesion is unencapsulated and infiltrates the bone extensively.

**407**

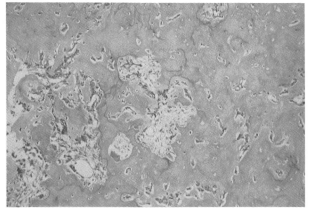

**408**

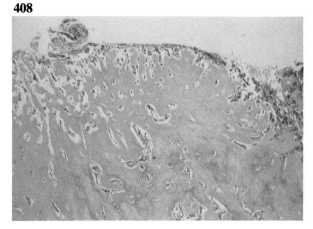

**407 Benign cementoblastoma.** There is a calcified tissue resembling bone but which is relatively acellular. Marked evidence of previous remodelling is usually seen, with formation of prominent reversal lines. The cells may exhibit atypia.

**408 Benign cementoblastoma.** At the periphery of the lesion there is usually a zone of uncalcified cementoid, corresponding to the radiolucent area separating the lesion from normal bone in a radiograph.

**409**

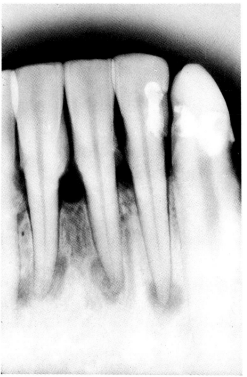

**410**

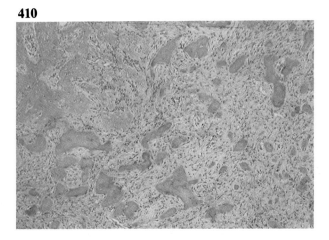

**409 Periapical cemental dysplasia.** This is usually seen related to the apices of the mandibular incisor teeth in middle-aged females. It commences as multiple radiolucencies which may be confused with periapical lesions. These gradually become radiopaque and usually remain symptomless.

**410 Periapical cemental dysplasia.** Histologically, there are foci of cementum-like particles and trabeculae of woven bone in a fibrous stroma. These gradually fuse together to form a solid area.

**411 Gigantiform cementoma** (diffuse osseous dysplasia). This is typically seen as multiple radiopaque foci in the jaws of middle-aged negro females, although, probably, it can be seen in most other races. Histologically, a mass of fused cementum is the main feature.

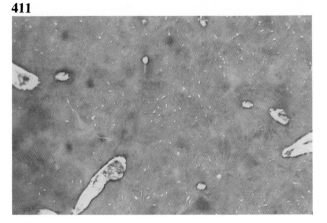

**411**

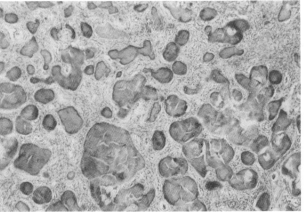

**412**

**412 'Cementifying fibroma'.** The lesion is circumscribed but not encapsulated, and is composed of multiple foci of cementicles in a fibrous connective tissue stroma. It is thought that the cementum-like masses fuse together to form a solid mass, but the lesion does not exhibit persistent growth. It is not to be confused with a histologically similar lesion which exhibits persistent growth. The latter is probably more appropriately regarded as an ossifying fibroma.

# 9 Diseases associated with microbiological agents

**413 Tuberculosis.** The typical histological appearance of the tubercle follicle is an aggregation of histiocytes called epithelioid cells, within which are found Langhans' type giant cells with nuclei at the periphery. Caseation necrosis occurs within the follicles soon after their formation.

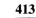
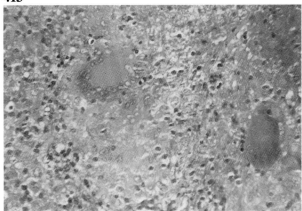

**414 Tuberculosis.** Higher power view of an area of caseation necrosis within a tuberculous lesion.

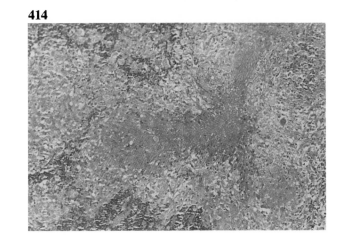

**415 Tuberculosis.** Acid-fast bacillus within the lesional tissue. (*Ziehl-Neelsen*)

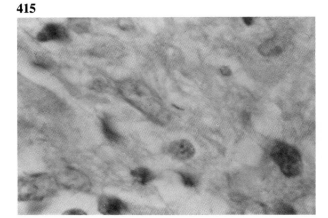

**416 Syphilis.** Focal aggregations of a predominantly plasma cell infiltrate around blood vessels are seen. Oral lesions which are not syphilitic frequently show this feature, and care must be taken not to over-diagnose lesions as syphilitic.

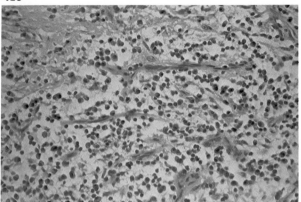

416

**417 Syphilis.** Endarteritis obliterans. The lumen of the blood vessel is severely narrowed by proliferation of the tunica intima.

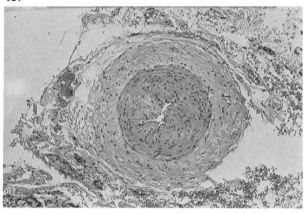

417

**418 Prenatal syphilis.** The classical presentation of prenatal syphilis is Hutchinsonian incisor teeth. The middle mamelon has failed to develop at the incisal edge, resulting in the formation of a notch.

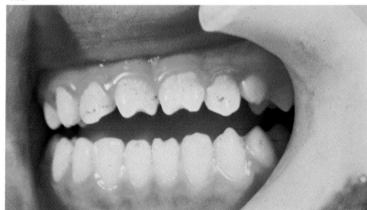

418

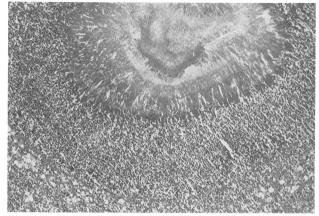

**419 Actinomycosis.** This is caused by a higher bacterium, Actinomyces israeli. The tissue changes associated with the organism are a combination of acute and chronic inflammation. The zone of acute inflammation is seen as a zone of polymorphonuclear leucocyte infiltration around the colony of actinomyces.

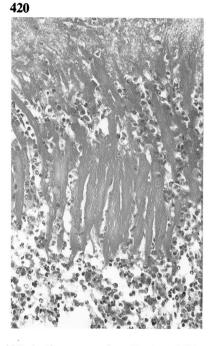

**420 Actinomycosis.** Eosinophilic clubs, which are Gram-negative are seen at the periphery; these are thought to be lipid material deposited around the filaments of actinomyces.

**421 Histoplasmosis.** The tissues are diffusely infiltrated with histiocytes with the causative organism, Histoplasma capsulatum, engulfed within the cytoplasm.

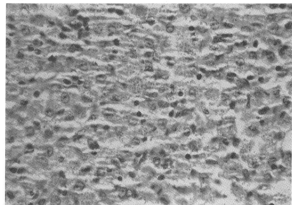

**422 Candidosis** (Candidiasis). The tissue changes in candidosis are variable. In the chronic hyperplastic form, the epithelium undergoes gross hyperplasia, with long and broad rete processes.

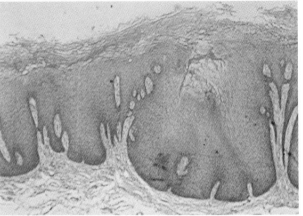

422

**423 Candidosis** (Candidiasis). Cellular atypia is seen within the deeper epithelial cells; increased mitotic activity is particularly prominent.

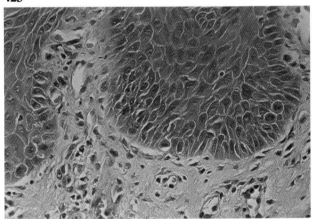

423

**424 Candidosis** (Candidiasis). The superficial layers of the epithelium which is usually parakeratotic, are diffusely infiltrated with polymorphonuclear leucocytes, sometimes even as microabscesses. Hyphae of Candida albicans can be demonstrated penetrating the superficial layers of epithelium. *(Periodic acid-Schiff)*

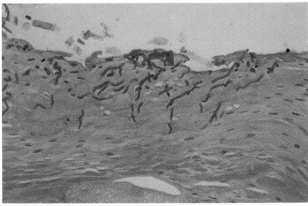

424

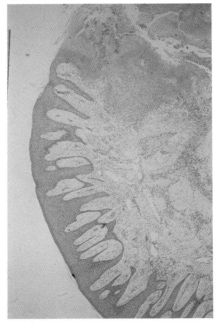

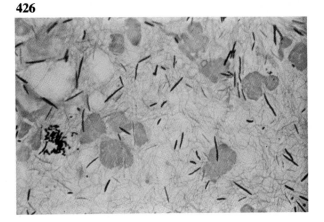

**426 Micro-organisms associated with acute ulcerative gingivitis.** A bacterial smear will reveal large numbers of two organisms, a spirochaete, Treponema vincenti, and a rod, Bacillus fusiformis. The role of these organisms in the causation of the disease has not been established. *(Gram)*

**425 Acute ulcerative gingivitis.** The interdental papilla is blunted and destroyed and the tissues are covered with a felted mass of micro-organisms. A diffuse zone of inflammation is seen beneath this area.

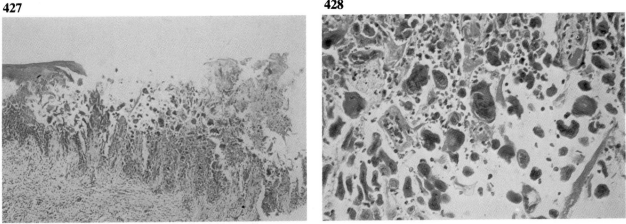

**427 and 428 Herpes simplex** (Primary herpetic gingivostomatitis). The oral lesions are vesicles which coalesce to form shallow ulcers. In histological examination of collapsed vesicles, an intra-epithelial vesicle with multinucleated epithelial giant cells is normally seen.

**429 Herpes simplex.** Exfoliative cytological smears from intact or recently ruptured vesicles will show the typical multinucleated giant cells. They are also seen, however, in herpes zoster and chicken pox vesicles.

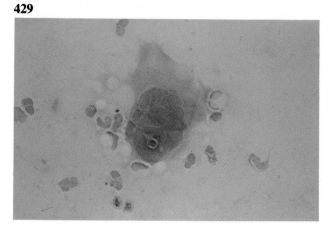

**430 Aspergillosis.** The fungus Aspergillus fumigata sometimes presents as a 'fungal ball' in the maxillary sinus. They apparently lie free within the antral cavity and do not penetrate the lining.

430

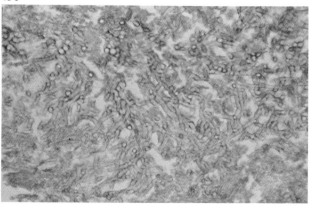

**431 Verruca vulgaris.** The common wart presents as a papilloma with multiple finger-like processes covered with a keratotic or parakeratotic stratified squamous epithelium. Vacuolated cells may be seen within the Stratum granulosum.

431

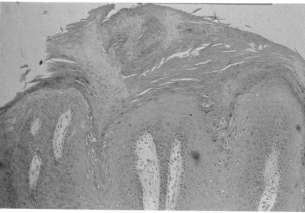

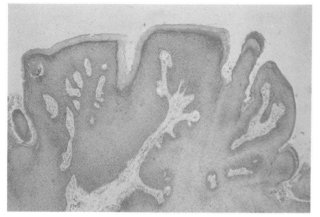

**432 Condyloma acuminatum.** The venereal wart, which is sexually transmitted, also presents as a papillomatous lesion.

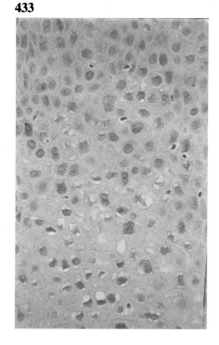

**433 Condyloma acuminatum.** Koilocytes (cells with a perinuclear halo) are seen within the prickle-cell layer and it is now accepted that they represent a cytopathic effect of the virus.

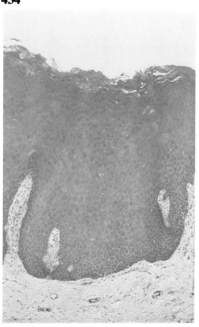

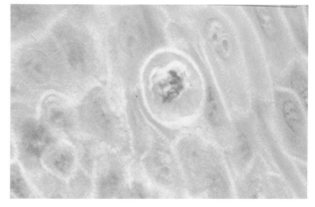

**435 Focal epithelial hyperplasia.** Higher power view of cells within the stratum malpighi reveal the presence of cells in 'mitosoid degeneration'.

**434 Focal epithelial hyperplasia** (Heck's disease). This condition, which is thought to be induced by a papovavirus, presents as multiple papules on the oral mucosa. Histologically, they are seen as acanthotic parakeratinized stratified squamous epithelium on a corium that is essentially normal.

# 10 Pigmented lesions

**436 Melanotic macule.** This presents as a small pigmented area on the oral mucosa. Histologically, the basal layer is darkly pigmented in the region of the lesion. Occasional melanophages may be seen in the corium.

**436**

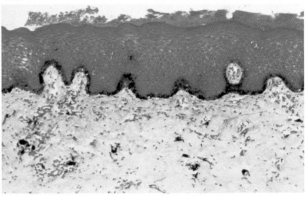

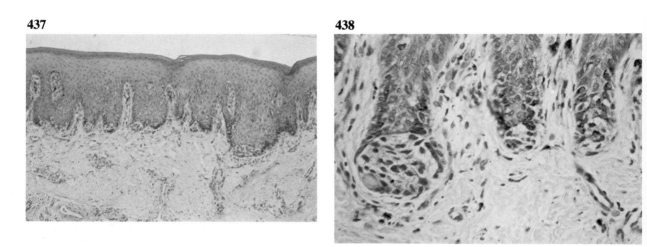

**437 and 438 Juctional naevus.** Well-circumscribed naevus cell nests are present in the basal region of the epithelium.

Figure **438** shows a higher power view of the naevus cell nests.

**439**

**440**

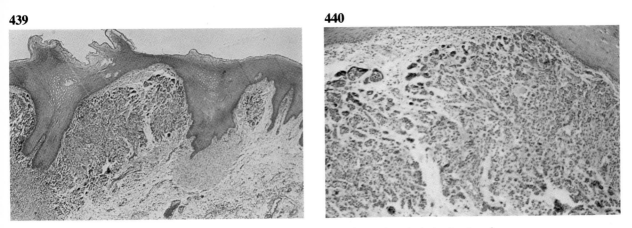

**439 and 440 Intradermal naevus.** The foci of naevus cells are situated entirely in the dermis.

**441**

**442**

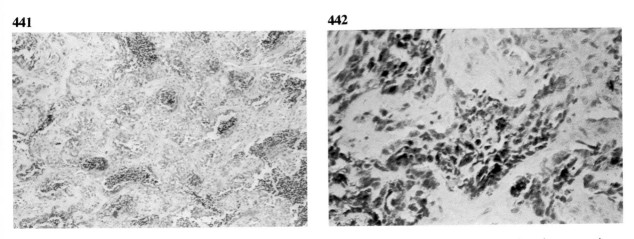

**441 and 442 Melanotic neuroectodermal tumour of infancy.** This usually presents as a melanotic tumour in infants 6 to 12 months old. The maxillary alveolus is the usual site and, despite the alarming clinical appearances, most reported cases are benign. Histologically, there are two cell types, epithelial-like cells containing melanin, and lymphocyte-like cells.

Figure **442** shows a higher power view of the pigmented cells in the epithelial islands.

**443 Malignant melanoma.** A darkly pigmented tumour mass is present in the palate of this 35-year-old man.

**443**

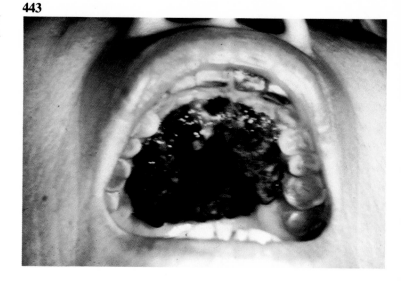

**444**

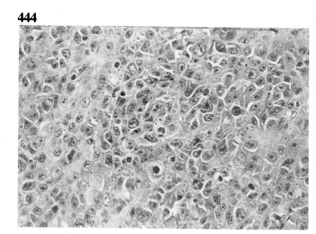

**445**

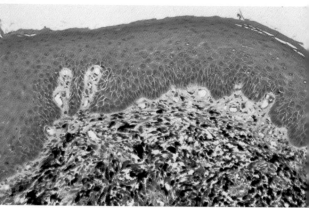

**444 Malignant melanoma.** The tumour cells exhibit marked pleomorphism and hyperchromatism. Nuclei with prominent nucleoli are marked. Relatively few cells contain the pigment.

**445 Malignant melanoma.** The tumour cells here are heavily pigmented with melanin; cellular detail has been obscured.

**446 Bismuth pigmentation.** Therapeutic administration of heavy metallic salts may result in the formation of lines in the gingiva. Histologically, these are seen as irregular black particles of sulphide of the metallic salt in the lamina propria close to the crevicular epithelium.

**446**

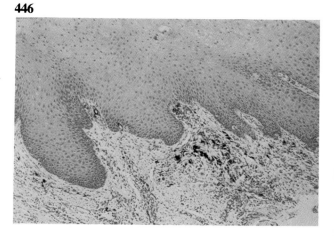

# 11 Granulomatous lesions

**447 Sarcoidosis.** In this disorder of uncertain origin, multiple systems of the body are involved. The oral manifestations include a diffuse enlargement of the gingivae and multiple soft tissue lumps on various parts of the oral mucosa. Multiple non-caseating tuberculoid foci are seen in the gingiva.

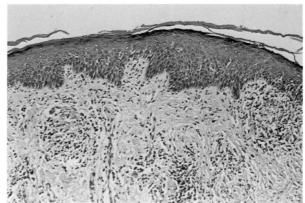

**448 Sarcoidosis.** Multiple foci of epithelioid cells which make up the tuberculoid follicles together with Langhans' type giant cells are seen within sarcoid lesions. Rarely, caseation may be visible within the follicles.

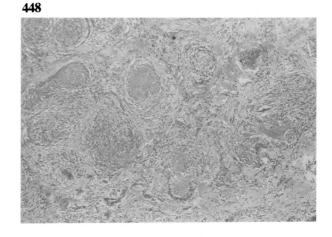

**449 Sarcoidosis.** A diffuse cervical lymphadenopathy should alert the clinician to the possibility of sarcoidosis.

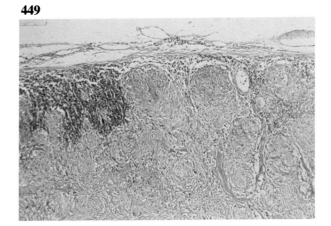

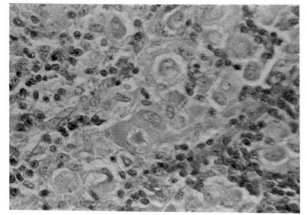

**450 Sarcoidosis.** Within the cytoplasm of the Langhans' type giant cells 'asteroid bodies' may be seen. Their nature is still debated. A recent study suggests that they may be related to the cell spindle.

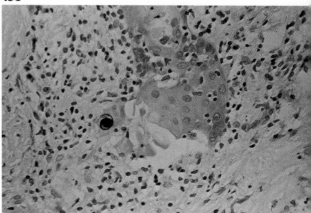

**451 Sarcoidosis.** Schaumann bodies, which are laminated calcified bodies, also may be seen within the cytoplasm of the giant cells.

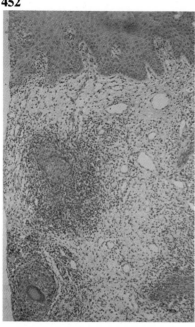

**452 Crohn's disease.** Non-caseating tuberculoid follicles, similar in appearance to those seen in sarcoidosis, are apparent in Crohn's disease. This is a disorder of unknown aetiology affecting primarily the gastro-intestinal tract, and oral lesions clinically manifesting as 'cobblestone mucosa' may be the presenting sign.

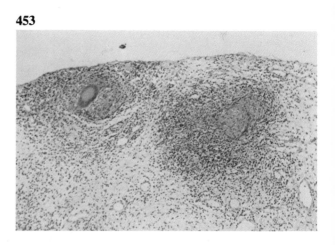

**453 Crohn's disease.** Non-caseating tuberculoid foci in an oedematous connective tissue stroma. Similar foci appear in 'cheilitis granulomatosa', and in Melkersson–Rosenthal syndrome.

**454 'Chronic periosteitis'.** In this inflammatory lesion, presenting classically in edentulous patients with complete dentures, multiple discharging sinuses may be present in the mouth. In addition to diffuse aggregations of inflammatory cells of both acute and chronic type, foci of histiocytes and giant cells are associated with eosinophilic ring-like structures. These have been referred to as 'pulse granulomas' but are composed of degenerate collagen fibres.

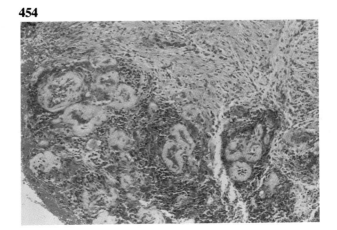

454

**455 Wegener's granulomatosis.** This is a condition which may affect the upper respiratory tract, terminating with renal complications. Oral lesions include a diffuse granular gingivitis and clinical appearances of a destructive lesion often diagnosed as a midline lethal granuloma. Histologically, in addition to a vasculitis, giant cells may be prominent in the inflammatory cell infiltrate.

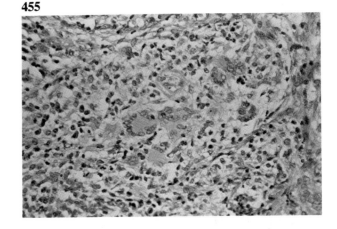

455

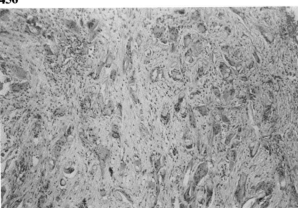

456

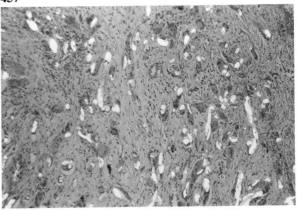

457

**456 Foreign body granuloma.** Foreign bodies which are introduced into the oral tissues may provoke a giant cell reaction mimicking a 'giant cell' lesion.

**457 Foreign body granuloma.** Under polarised light, the doubly-refractile or birefringent foreign material can be seen clearly within the cytoplasm of the foreign body giant cells.

# 12 Non-neoplastic salivary gland diseases

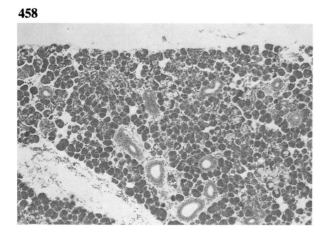

**458 Serous salivary gland lobules.** These appear in the parotid and submandibular glands, although they may be seen in some of the minor glands of the mouth.

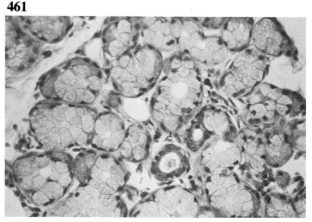

**459 Serous cells and striated ducts.** The serous cells contain large numbers of zymogen granules and the striated ducts show longitudinal striations in the cytoplasm.

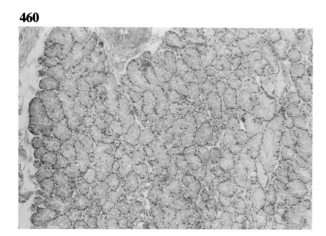

**460 Mucous salivary gland lobules.** The sublingual gland and the palatal glands consist entirely of mucous lobules. The submandibular gland contains both mucous and serous lobules.

Hypertrophy of mucous glands of the palate may present as a swelling simulating a salivary gland tumour. Histological examination, however, reveals that it is composed of normal mucous glands which may be enlarged.

**461 Mixed salivary gland lobules.** These contain a mixture of mucous and serous glands, often with a cap of serous cells on mucous secreting cells.

**462**

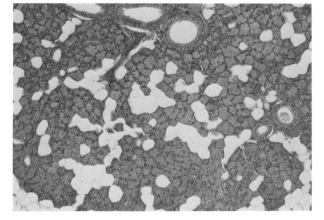

**462 Sialosis.** This condition presents as bilateral enlargement of the parotid glands, usually in patients with a history of systemic disease, such as diabetes mellitus. The serous cells appear enlarged with loss of granules. There is extensive replacement of the glandular parenchyma by adipose tissue.

**463**

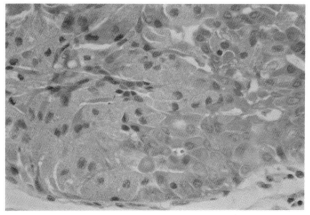

**463 Oncocytosis.** Oncocytes are parenchymal cells with eosinophilic granules in the cytoplasm which are shown to be mitochondria at the ultrastructural level. They are seen in the ductal cells, but groups of acini may also undergo this change, probably increasing in frequency with advancing years.

**464**

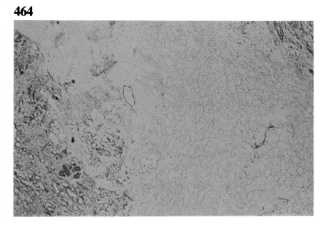

**464 Necrotising sialometaplasia.** This condition could be mistaken for a salivary gland neoplasm, as it may present as an ulcerated palatal swelling. Histologically, there are areas in which structure has been destroyed with the appearance of an infarct.

**465**

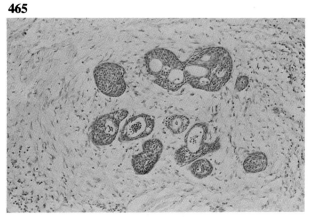

**465 Necrotising sialometaplasia.** Other areas show squamous metaplasia of the ducts which may mimic the appearance of a mucoepidermoid tumour.

**466 Sialoadenitis.** The secretory elements in the acini are decreased with a relative increase in ductal structures. Inter- and intra-lobular fibrosis may be prominent and chronic inflammatory cell infiltration of the lobules may be diffuse or focal.

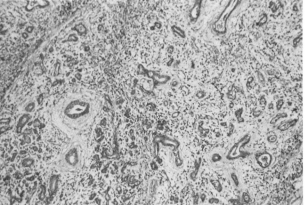

**467 Sialoadenitis.**

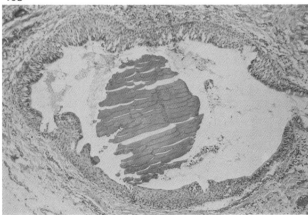

**468 Sialithiasis.** A salivary calculus may be seen within the duct of this minor salivary gland.

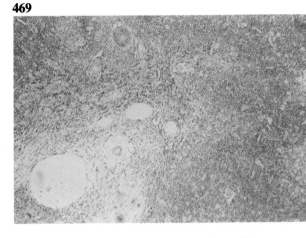

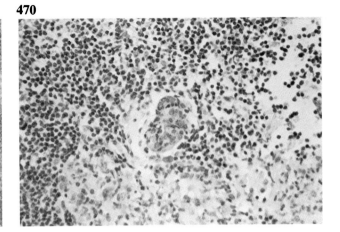

**469 Sjögren's syndrome.** The major salivary glands show a replacement of the gland parenchyma by lymphoid tissue, with proliferation of 'epimyoepithelial islands'.

**470 Sjögren's syndrome.** Higher power view of the lymphoid replacement and an 'epimyoepithelial island'.

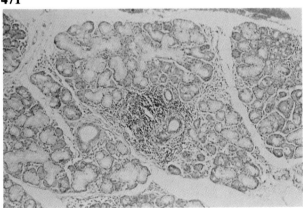

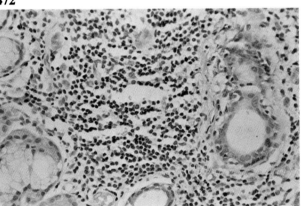

**471 Sjögren's syndrome** (labial gland biopsy). Lobules of labial glands removed show focal accumulations of lymphocytes within the lobules. The importance of this technique in the diagnosis of Sjögren's syndrome has diminished in recent years.

**472 Sjögren's syndrome** (labial gland biopsy). Higher power view of the focal accumulations of lymphocytes in the labial gland lobules.

**473**

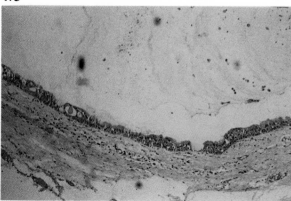

**474**

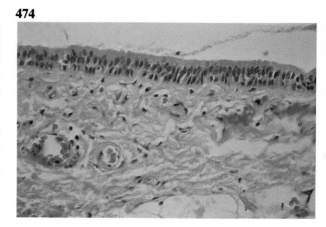

**473 Mucous retention cyst.** In the genuine mucous retention cyst there is an epithelial lining which is usually twin-layered ductal epithelium. The cyst cavity is filled with mucin and inflammatory cells are not common.

**474** Higher power view of the twin-layered ductal epithelium.

**475**

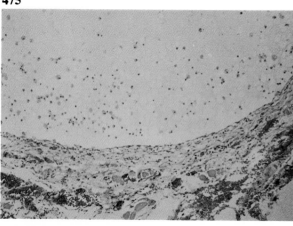

**476**

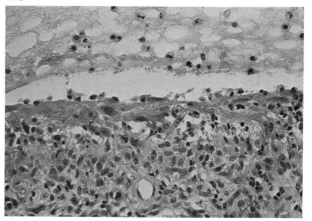

**475 Mucous extravasation cyst.** The mucous extravasation cyst is more common than the mucous retention cyst. It has a lining of condensed fibroblasts and macrophages and, within the cavity filled with a mucinous fluid, there are many mucinophages and polymorphonuclear leucocytes.

**476** Higher power view of the lining of condensed fibroblasts and macrophages.

# Bibliography

Batsakis, J. G. (1979). *Tumours of the head and neck.* (2nd ed.) Williams and Wilkins, Baltimore.

Berkovitz, B.K.B., Moxham, G.J. and Newman, H.N. (edits.) (1982). *The periodontal ligament in health and disease.* Pergamon, Oxford.

Brannstrom, M. (1981). *Dentine and pulp in restorative dentistry.* Dental Therapeutics AB, Nacka, Sweden.

Cohen, B. and Kramer, I. R. H. (edits.) (1976). *Scientific foundations of dentistry.* Heinemann, London.

Gorlin, R. J., Pindborg, J. J. and Cohen, M. M. Jnr. (1976). *Syndromes of the head and neck.* (2nd ed.) McGraw Hill, New York.

Jones, J. H. and Mason, D. K. (edits.) (1980). *Oral manifestations of systemic disease.* Saunders, London.

Lucas, R. B. (1984). *Pathology of tumours of the oral tissues.* (4th ed.) Churchill Livingstone, London.

Mackenzie, I. C., Dabelsteen, E. and Squire, C. (edits.) (1980). *Oral precancer.* Iowa University Press.

Pindborg, J. J. (1980). *Oral cancer and precancer.* Wright, Bristol.

Pindborg, J. J. (1980). *Atlas of diseases of the oral mucosa.* (3rd ed.) Munksgaard, Copenhagen.

Pindborg, J. J. and Hjørting-Hansen, E. (1974). *Atlas of diseases of the jaws.* Munksgaard, Copenhagen.

Pindborg, J. J. and Kramer, I. R. H. (1972). *Histological typing of odontogenic tumours, jaw cysts and allied lesions.* W.H.O., Geneva.

Shafer, W. G., Hine, M. K. and Levy, B. (1983). *Textbook of oral pathology.* (4th ed.) Saunders, Philadelphia.

Shear, M. (1983). *Cysts of the oral regions.* (2nd ed.) Wright, Bristol.

Silverstone, L., Johnson, N. W., Hardie, J. M. and Williams, R. D. (1981). *Dental caries.* Macmillan, London.

Stewart, R. D. and Prescott, G. H. (edits.) (1976). *Oral facial genetics.* Mosby, St Louis.

Thackray, A. C. and Lucas, R. B. (1979). *Tumours of the major salivary glands.* Armed Forces Institute of Pathology, Washington.

W.H.O. Collaborating Centre for Oral Precancerous Lesions, Copenhagen. (1978). Definition of leukoplakia and related lesions: an aid to studies on oral precancer. *Oral Surg.* **46;** 518-539.

Wright, D. H. and Isaacson, P. G. (1983). *Biopsy pathology of the lymphoreticular system.* Chapman and Hall, London.

# Index

# Index

Numbers refer to illustrations.